Susannah James

Lose Weight FAST With

Fat Blasting Smoothies

1st Edition

Lose Weight FAST With Fat Blasting Smoothies

1st Edition

First published 2017

Published by Lionheart Publishing

Copyright © 2016 Lionheart Publishing

Notice of Liability

A great deal of effort has gone into ensuring that the content of this book is both accurate and up to date. However, Lionheart Publishing and the author will not be held liable for any loss or damage from the use of the information herein

Trademarks

All trademarks are acknowledged as belonging to their respective companies

ISBN-13: 978-1977564481

ISBN-10: 1977564488

Contents

Chapter 1 - Before You Start

Chapter 2 – Smoothies For Losing Weight

Chapter 3 – Smoothies to Get You Going

Chapter 8 – Smoothies That Keep Your Heart Healthy

Chapter 9 – Smoothies For the Immune System

Chapter 10 – Smoothies For Diabetics

Chapter 11 – Smoothies For Extra Energy

Chapter 12 – Smoothies For Bones & Teeth

Chapter 13 – Smoothies For General Good Health

Nutrition Tables Weight Conversion Tables

CHAPTER 1

Before You Start

Chapter One is an introduction to the subject of smoothies. We start by looking at the various reasons people take these drinks and why they are so popular, i.e. the health benefits they offer.

For example, smoothies provide an excellent way of losing weight and many people get into them for just this reason. We explain how to incorporate smoothies into the various types of diet plan.

We also show you what you should be looking for when buying a blender, and give you some handy blending tips that will ensure your smoothies are perfect everytime.

Introduction

Recent years have seen people becoming aware of just how important their diet is. Not so long ago, animal fat was considered to be the number one cause of the obesity epidemic in western countries and, accordingly, diet plans at the time focused on eliminating these fats. Then the focus switched to sugar as people began to realize how widespread the use of it was, not just in the obvious such as cakes, cookies, etc but also in soups, drinks, sauces and a multitude of other types of food.

One result of the awareness of the dangers of excessive fat and sugar has been the rise of smoothies and juicing amongst health-concious people. Needless to say, the food industry has not been slow to catch on – commercially produced smoothies and juices are now available and are marketed as being healthy and as a way of losing weight. Do not be deceived – these products usually have a high sugar content (with the attendant high level of calories) and contain all the usual preservatives and additives.

For the health-concious individual, there is only one option – make your own. By doing so, you can ensure they contain only fresh ingredients, are created exactly to your taste, and do not contain preservatives. Furthermore, you can create smoothies for a variety of purposes. These include weight loss, beauty, cognitive function, the prevention/treatment of specific diseases, ailments such as diabetes and keeping the advance of old age at bay.

In chapters 1-13, you will discover a wide range of smoothie recipes that can be enjoyed simply as part of a healthy diet, or to achieve specific goals such as those mentioned above.

The Benefits of Smoothies

Smoothies are created almost exclusively from vegetables, fruits, seeds and nuts. This fact alone makes them inherently healthy - no artery-clogging animal fats and very little waistline-expanding sugar. More specific benefits include:

Your daily ration of fruit and vegetables - getting the daily recommendation of fruit and vegetables can be a challenge for people who lead busy lives. Incorporating them into a smoothie is an easy way of way of ensuring you get your daily nutritional needs.

Convenience - making smoothies is quicker than preparing a meal, leaving more time for other activities. You can also drink a smoothie at any time; not just at meal times. So if you don't have time for breakfast, simply take it with you and have it later on.

Kids love them - getting your kids to eat healthy foods can be hard. Smoothies provide an answer as most kids love the taste of a creamy smoothie. You can hide vegetables in your kid's smoothies that they don't like and would never eat by choice.

Weight loss - drinking smoothies is an excellent way of losing weight. They can provide all the essential vitamins and minerals your body needs while eliminating the unwanted fats and sugars.

Fibre - the fruits and vegetables that comprise your smoothies are packed with fibre. Not only does a high fibre intake protect against heart disease, type 2 diabetes and bowel cancer, it also slows down digestion and helps to keep blood sugar at a healthy level.

Protein - another vital dietary requirement, protein can be incorporated into smoothies by adding nut butters such as peanut butter. A good alternative is avocado, which has a high protein content.

cont'd

Detoxification - detoxification is about cleaning and nourishing the body from the inside out. By removing and eliminating toxins, then feeding your body with healthy nutrients, detoxification can not only protect you from disease but also enable you to maintain optimum health. Smoothies provide the ideal way to do this.

Refuelling - two crucial elements required to help your body recover after strenuous exertion, are protein for muscle repair and carbohydrates to replenish your energy levels. A smoothie containing both provides a great way of recuperating and also hydrating yourself at the same time.

The body beautiful - a plentiful supply of the vitamins and minerals found in fruits and vegetables is essential for keeping hair, skin and nails looking good.

A good nights sleep - regular consumption of health-giving smoothies is guaranteed to help you sleep better at night. Don't forget, if you don't sleep properly, you will never be healthy regardless of what you eat and drink.

Brain power - without the necessary nutrients, your brain cannot function at its best. Giving it what it needs in the form of smoothies will improve cognition, memory and your ability to focus - brain fog will be a thing of the past.

Fun - making smoothies needn't be a chore. By altering the recipes in this book, or experimenting to create your own, making smoothies can be a creative and enjoyable pastime.

Smoothies as Part of a Diet Plan

Eating a healthy balanced diet is crucial in reducing the risk of getting heart disease and any of the various forms of cancer. It also ensures you maintain a healthy weight and engenders general well-being.

A healthy and balanced diet plan involves eating six main types of food. In no particular order, these are:

Protein - this is found in meat, fish, dairy produce, nuts and some types of vegetable.

Carbohydrates - the main source of carbohydrates are sugar, dried fruit, cereals, cookies & cakes, flour, jams & preserves, bread, pasta and potatoes.

Calcium - calcium is required for good bone health and is found in dairy products such as cheese and milk.

Omega-3 oil - this provides essential fatty acids that support, among other things, the maintenance of vision and brain function. It is found in nuts and oily fish such as tuna and salmon.

Fibre - fibre is crucial for digestive health and the prevention of heart disease, certain cancers and diabetes. Foods rich in fibre include fruits, vegetables, beans and nuts.

In this book you will find a number of smoothie recipes that incorporate all of the above foods. These smoothies provide you with all the nutrients necessary to maintain perfect health. Diet, however, is not always about maintaining general good health. Many diet plans are followed for specific reasons such as losing weight, lowering cholesterol levels, controlling diabetes and detoxifying the body.

cont'd

Smoothies can complement these diet plans, or even replace them completely. For example:

Low Carbohydrate Diets

Low carb-diets are essential for people with diabetes, who have to keep the glucose in their blood at a certain level. Smoothies made mainly from fruit and vegetables fit the bill here as we see on pages 102-110

Weight Loss Diets

Fats and carbohydrates are the enemy with regard to body weight. It is very easy to make smoothies that have minimal quantities of both, or even none, and regular consumption of them will shift those stubborn pounds fast. You will find many suitable weight-loss smoothie recipes on pages 20-30.

High Protein Diets

There are occasions when extra protein is required. For example, childhood/adolescence (growth), pregnancy, lactation, intense strength and endurance training, and certain illnesses. The elderly may also need additional amounts of protein.

High Fibre Diets

Including enough fibre in our diets is essential primarily for healthy bowel function. It also reduces the risk of coronary heart disease, colon cancer, diabetes and obesity. However, it is a fact that many people in the western world don't have anything like enough fibre in their diets.

Blending versus Juicing

A common question is what is the difference between juicing and blending? Now, you might think the difference is obvious - but there is actually a lot of confusion about this.

Juicing

Juicing is a process which extracts the water and nutrients from food and discards the fibre. Without the fibre, your digestive system doesn't have to break down the food and so can absorb the nutrients quickly. As as a result, the nutrients are readily available to the body, and in much larger quantities than if you were to eat the food, whatever it is, whole.

Freshly squeezed vegetable juices form part of most healing and detoxification programs because they are so nutrient-rich and nourish and restore the body at a cellular level.

Blending (Smoothies)

Unlike juices, blended smoothies can contain the entire fruit or vegetable, including the fibre. Because of this, the nutrients are released into the bloodstream more slowly and evenly, thus avoiding spikes in blood sugar levels. The presence of the fibre also makes the smoothie more filling, and so more likely to keep you satisfied until your next meal.

This issue of fibre is an important one. Because of the lack of it, green juices, particularly when you are doing extended juice detoxification programs, can actually damage your health. Drinking nothing but juice can deliver an unhealthy dose of rapidly absorbed sugar into your bloodstream.

Blenders are cheap - you may already have one. Juicing machines on the other hand, are more complex and good ones are expensive.

Buying a Blender

When buying a blender, the following factors should be taken into account:

- Counter-top or immersion - counter-top blenders are made for countertops with a large jar attached to a stand on which are the blender controls. Immersion blenders are small hand-held devices with a rotating blade at the end. The counter-top type is the one you want ideally

- Power - a wide range of blenders are available with different power ratings. Go for one with a rating of 500 watts or above

- Controls - some blenders come with manual speed control and may only provide one speed. Better blenders will offer variable speed control. The most expensive blenders are microprocessor controlled and offer a range of blending options. Also well worth having is a pulse function

- Blade assembly - blending can be a messy business so we recommend you get a blender that has easy-to-remove stainless steel blades

- Blender jar - blender jars come in plastic, glass and stainless steel. Each has its pros and cons. For example, glass (the recommended option) is easy to maintain, and is transparent so you can easily see when the smoothie is ready. They are, however, easy to break. You may also want to consider the jar's capacity

- Ice blade - some blenders come with an ice-crushing blade that lets you make ice-cold smoothies (handy in summer)

Note: don't buy a food processor by mistake. These devices are designed for use with solid foods, not liquids as with smoothies.

Blending Tips

Having purchased your blender, you are now ready to get down to business. Observation of the following tips will ensure your smoothies are perfect every time:

- Fix the blender's blades into position *before* you start adding the ingredients

- Be sure to remove all fruit stones - these can damage the blender's blades

- Cut your ingredients into chunks before adding them to the blender. All blenders work best with certain chunk sizes and you may need to experiment to find the optimal size for your machine

- When ice is being used in a smoothie, always add it last. You may, otherwise, over-blend the ice thus making the smoothie watery. A different option if you want a cold smoothie is to use frozen fruit rather than fresh fruit

- Make sure the lid is securely in place before switching the blender on. The mess these devices can create has to be seen to be believed

- Instead of using tap water to make your ice cubes, use coconut water. Doing this will add valuable nutrients such as potassium and magnesium

- It's better to add too little liquid rather than too much. You can always add more if necessary

- Don't overfill the blender - leave room for expansion by leaving at least a third empty. Otherwise, you may have some cleaning up to do!

cont'd

- If you have a multi-speed or variable speed blender, increase the speed in stages. This helps to blend the ingredients evenly and results in a smoother smoothie

- Don't use sugar to sweeten your smoothies. Instead, add pear juice, very ripe bananas, grape juice, apple juice, pomegranate juice, pitted dates; or a small amount of agave syrup, maple syrup or honey

- Organically grown produce almost always has more flavour and nutrients than conventionally farmed fruit. Therefore, whenever possible, use organic fruits and vegetables

- For an ultra-creamy smoothie, try adding a small piece of avocado, a couple of spoons of oatmeal, or a spoonful or two of coconut oil

- Leafy greens should be put in the blender first. This stops them floating at the top and not being blended properly

- Having made a smoothie, ideally, you should drink it within 30 minutes or so. If you leave it longer, oxidation may take place and destroy some of the nutrients. Furthermore, the ingredients may separate

- Smoothies provide you with the perfect opportunity to try out the various 'superfoods' such as avocados, blueberries, goji berries, maca, cacao, etc

Using This Book

The smoothie recipes in this book are laid out by type, with each chapter containing recipes created for a specific purpose. In chapter 13, we show you a number of smoothies that have been created for overall good health.

Measures

All ingredient quantities are specified in standard U.S. measures, i.e. cups and spoons. For non-american readers, we include conversion charts - see page 146.

Fruit and vegetables come in all shapes and sizes. Please note that when we specify an item, we mean an item of medium size (unless stated otherwise).

All quantities given are approximate - they are not written in stone. Feel free to add more or less of any ingredient if you so wish; or indeed, add different ones and leave others out.

Create Your Own

Given the huge range of ingredients available, there is absolutely no limit to the potential smoothie combinations. While we encourage you to try the recipes detailed in the book - they are all tried and tested - why stop there? Also, smoothies aren't just about health; many people enjoy the process of creating them just as much as they do consuming them.

Just in case you do decide to have a go yourself, we have listed the most commonly used ingredients on pages 141-145. Many people of course, will want or need, to create smoothies for a specific purpose. To help them do so, we have included the important nutritional values for all of the ingredients.

Purpose

When creating smoothies, don't lose sight of why you're creating

cont'd

them in the first place. It's a fact that many smoothies, usually the ones containing vegetables, can taste a bit 'odd'. Remember, it's your health that's the important thing, whether or not you actually enjoy drinking the thing is secondary.

This raises another issue - that of consistency. A smoothie is a drink and so will have a certain consistency. Some people like them thick and creamy, others prefer them thin and watery. If any of our recipes are not to your liking in this respect, just add more liquid to thin them out, or add more fruit/vegetables to make them thicker. Another way is to add some ice to the mix and blend it again.

Smoothies for Diabetics

People with type 1 diabetes need to match their carbohydrate intake with their insulin dose. To help with this, every one of our recipes clearly shows the carbohydrate content.

CHAPTER 2

Smoothies For Losing Weight

The two main problems with dieting to lose weight are you have to eat less, which leaves you feeling hungry, and by eating less, you may not get enough of the essential nutrients that your body needs to function properly. Smoothies provide the perfect solution to both of these issues. With regard to feeling hungry, this happens because you aren't getting enough of the fibre that fills you up. Smoothies comprised largely of fibre-rich fruit and vegetables eliminates this. Add some other ingredients to provide the required nutrients and you'll be hitting your weight loss target before you know it.

Melon and Lime Cocktail

A zingy and highly refreshing smoothie that combines the great tastes of watermelon and lime. The addition of mint gives it a cocktail feel.

Ingredients
1 1/2 cups chopped watermelon
1/2 lime
4 mint leaves
1/2 cup crushed ice

Preparation
Any type of watermelon will work but honeydew is ideal. Peel the lime and add it to the rest of the ingredients in the blender. Add the ice last and blend until smooth.

Nutrition
Calories – 77g
Fibre – 2.5g
Fat – 0g
Protein – 2g
Carbohydrate – 20g

Ingredient Spotlight - Watermelon

The main constituent of watermelon is water – 92 percent. It is, however, loaded with nutrients. These include vitamins A, B6 and C, lycopene, antioxidants and amino acids.

Furthermore, it is fat-free and has only 45 calories per cup. It has anti-inflammatory properties, provides a high level of fibre for healthy digestion, vitamin A for skin and hair, and protects against cancer thanks to its antioxidants (lycopene, in particular, is thought to be effective against prostate cancer).

Tomato Head

This is a rich tasting smoothie that will slip down a treat. Packed with fibre from the radish, tomato, pepper, and celery, it will keep you feeling full and free from hunger pangs.

Ingredients

1/2 cup radish

1 tomato

1 bell pepper

2 celery sticks

1 cup water

Preparation

Place all the ingredients in the blender. Then blend until nice and smooth.

Nutrition

Calories – 71g

Fibre – 5.5g

Fat – 0g

Protein – 4g

Carbohydrate – 19g

Ingredient Spotlight - Tomatoes

Tomatoes have a relatively high water content, which makes them a filling food. They also make your skin look great due to their beta-carotene content that helps protect skin against sun damage.

The lycopene in tomatoes also makes skin less sensitive to UV light damage - a leading cause of fine lines and wrinkles.

Raspberry Ripple

A sharp-tasting smoothie that will be perfect for quenching your thirst, while at the same time, being low in calories.

Ingredients
1 cup raspberries
1 kiwi
1/2 lime
1/2 cup crushed ice

Preparation
Peel the lime before adding to the blender. Then add the other ingredients and blend until smooth.

Nutrition
Calories – 116g
Fibre – 11g
Fat – 1.5g
Protein – 3g
Carbohydrate – 23g

Ingredient Spotlight - Raspberries

Cholesterol-free, low in fat and sodium, and with a modest 64 calories per cup, raspberries are an excellent food for dieters.

They contain high levels of vitamins and minerals needed for a number of body functions, such as bone development. Raspberries can also fight inflammatory conditions such as arthritis and gout.

The Energizer

Drink this one for an on-the-go breakfast, to refuel after a workout, or for a mid-afternoon energizer. Whichever, it's very low in calories and will have you shedding the pounds fast while, at the same time, keeping your energy levels high.

Ingredients
1 cup spinach
1 banana
1/2 cup unsweetened almond milk

Preparation
Add all the ingredients to the blender and blend until smooth. As with all leafy greens, put the spinach in the blender first.

Nutrition
Calories – 142g
Fibre – 4g
Fat – 1g
Protein – 3g
Carbohydrate – 41g

Ingredient Spotlight - Spinach

Spinach is well known for its nutritional qualities and has a remarkable ability to restore energy, increase vitality and improve the quality of the blood.

The primary reason for this is the fact that it is rich in iron. Iron plays a central role in the function of red blood cells, which help in transporting oxygen around the body during energy production and DNA synthesis.

Pumpkin Shake

A low-calorie, high-fibre smoothie that will be keep you feeling full and away from the food cupboard.

Ingredients

1 cup pumpkin
1 carrot
1/2 apple
1/2 cup unsweetened almond milk

Preparation

Cut the pumpkin, apple and carrot into chunks before adding to the blender with the almond milk. Blend until smooth.

Nutrition

Calories – 132g
Fibre – 5g
Fat – 0g
Protein – 1.5g
Carbohydrate – 30g

Ingredient Spotlight - Pumpkin

Very low in calories and containing no saturated fats or cholesterol, pumpkin is the perfect food to include in a calorie-controlled diet. An increasingly popular health food, it has a good amount of fibre that keeps you feeling full so you eat less overall. It is also rich in vitamin A, which promotes good vision and helps to maintain healthy skin.

Blueberry Bliss

The combination of antioxidant-packed spinach and blueberries, fibre-filled pear and alkalizing lemon, creates an absolute powerhouse of a smoothie.

Ingredients

1/2 cup blueberries

1/2 cup spinach

1 pear

1/2 lemon

1/2 cup coconut water

Preparation

Peel the lemon and add it and the other ingredients to the blender jar. Blend until smooth.

Nutrition

Calories – 172g

Fibre – 9g

Fat – 1g

Protein – 1.5g

Carbohydrate – 46g

Ingredient Spotlight - Blueberries

These delicious fruits are high in nutrients while, at the same time, having a very low calorific content - this makes them perfect for inclusion in a weight-loss diet.

Amongst the many health benefits provided by blueberries is that they help to prevent heart disease by keeping blood pressure low.

Go Bananas

You'll go bananas for this delicious smoothie. While it may have a few more calories, it will still help you lose weight and, at the same time, help to keep your skin nice and smooth.

Ingredients

1 banana
1/2 cup strawberries
1/2 cup blueberries
1 tablespoon almond butter
1/2 cup almond milk

Preparation

Add the ingredients to the blender and blend until smooth. Raspberries or cranberries can be substituted for the strawberries.

Nutrition

Calories – 302g
Fibre – 7g
Fat – 12.5g
Protein – 6.5g
Carbohydrate – 54g

Ingredient Spotlight - Bananas

Bananas are one of the healthiest foods you can eat. Amongst other things, they keep your bowels healthy, provide nutrients that regulate heart rhythm, and have vitamin compounds important for eye health. They are naturally free of fats and cholesterol.

With regard to weight loss, a medium banana has a negligible 105 calories but a whopping three grams of fibre that keeps you feeling full and helps get you through the day without snacking.

Moody Blues

This delicious smoothie combines the health giving properties of blueberries and ginger with the zinginess of lime for a sharp and refreshing drink that is very low in calories.

Ingredients
1 cup blueberries
1 inch piece of root ginger
1 lime
2 or 3 ice cubes

Preparation
Add all the ingredients to the blender, with the ice going in last, and blend until smooth.

Nutrition
Calories – 106g
Fibre – 7.5g
Fat – 0.5g
Protein – 1.5g
Carbohydrate – 30g

Ingredient Spotlight - Ginger

Ginger has a long history of use for relieving digestive problems such as nausea, loss of appetite, motion sickness and pain. Pregnant women experiencing morning sickness can safely use ginger to relieve nausea and vomiting.

During cold weather, taking ginger is good way to keep warm. It is diaphoretic, which means that it promotes sweating by working to warm the body from within.

Lean, Mean and Green

Cabbage and spinach are well known as excellent foods to include in a diet. Apples keep the doctor away, or so they say! – they certainly give this smoothie a nice taste. Add a kiwi for good measure and you have a very pleasant low-calorie smoothie.

Ingredients

1/2 cup cabbage

1/2 cup spinach

1/2 apple

1 kiwi

1 cup water

Preparation

Blend the water, cabbage and spinach first. Then add the apple and kiwi and blend again until smooth

Nutrition

Calories – 104g

Fibre – 6g

Fat – 1g

Protein – 2g

Carbohydrate – 25g

Ingredient Spotlight - Cabbage

Cabbage is an abundant source of vitamin C, which reduces the free radicals in your body that are one of the fundamental causes of premature aging.

It is also very helpful with regard to ulcers, certain cancers, depression, boosting the immune system, and providing protection against coughs and colds.

Fruit Fromage

The three main ingredients in this one are pineapple, grapefruit, and strawberry. These combine to produce a smoothie that is as delicious as it is healthy.

Ingredients

1/2 grapefruit
1/2 cup pineapple
1/2 cup strawberries
1/2 cup low-fat yoghurt
3/4 cup crushed ice

Preparation

Peel the grapefruit and cut it into chunks. Do the same with the pineapple if it is a fresh whole pineapple. Then place all the ingredients in the blender with the ice going in last. Then blend.

Nutrition

Calories – 168g
Fibre – 4g
Fat – 1.5g
Protein – 5g
Carbohydrate – 35g

Ingredient Spotlight - Grapefruit

Grapefruit contains a wide assortment of vitamins and minerals, one of the most important being potassium - this is a major constituent of the body's cells and fluids. It is also rich in vitamins, particularly A and C.

Other nutrients found in grapefruit include folate, thiamin, calcium and magnesium.

Pearfect

Get your day off to the perfect start with this pear and banana combo. High in that all-important vitamin C, it also has plenty of fibre, which promotes digestion and bowel health.

Ingredients

2 pears
1 banana
1/2 inch piece of root ginger
1/2 cup low-fat milk
Pinch of cinnamon or nutmeg

Preparation

Place all the ingredients in the blender and blend until smooth. Finish by adding a sprinkle of cinnamon or nutmeg.

Nutrition

Calories – 355g
Fibre – 14g
Fat – 2g
Protein – 6.5g
Carbohydrate – 85g

Ingredient Spotlight - Pears

Pears are rich in antioxidants, flavonoids and fibre, and pack all these nutrients in a fat- and cholesterol-free, 96 calorie package.

They also have a high pectin content, which helps to lower cholesterol levels. Pectin is diuretic and has a mild laxative.

CHAPTER 3

Smoothies to Get You Going

In this chapter, we look at smoothies suitable for starting the day with, i.e. breakfast. Many people skip breakfast completely and they do so for a number of reasons, one of which is that they think it helps them lose weight. Another is so-called lack of time. However, they are doing themselves no favours at all as, after eight hours or so without being topped up with a new supply of nutrients, the body starts to run out. The result is that it slows down – tiredness sets in more quickly, mental clarity decreases and general health is adversely affected. Smoothies are the answer. Quick to make and consume, a well crafted smoothie will provide all the nutrients necessary to get the system going, and keep it going, until the next meal.

Chocoholic

A perfect start to the day is guaranteed with this absolutely delicious chocolate and raspberry smoothie. Not only does it give you a healthy dose of vitamins and antioxidants, you get a protein boost to get your day started on the right foot.

Ingredients

1 cup spinach

1 cup raspberries

1 tablespoon cacao powder

1 tablespoon protein powder

Preparation

Place the spinach in the blender first, add the other ingredients and then blend until smooth.

Nutrition

Calories – 138g

Fibre – 12g

Fat – 4g

Protein – 13g

Carbohydrate – 22g

Ingredient Spotlight - Protein Powder

Our bodies use protein for the production of muscles, hormones, enzymes, immune-system components and much more. Given how important it is, it is always a good idea to get some inside you before your day begins.

Protein powder is an easy way to do this. It is made from milk and contains all nine essential amino acids. The type we recommend is whey protein powder.

Kale and Grape

The combination of kale, grapes and almond milk makes a sweet and refreshing breakfast smoothie.

Ingredients

1 cup grapes
1 cup kale
1/2 cup unsweetened almond milk

Preparation

Place the ingredients in the blender and blend until smooth. Red, green or black grapes can be used. You can also add one tablespoon of protein powder if you wish.

Nutrition

Calories – 173g
Fibre – 2g
Fat – 2g
Protein – 2g
Carbohydrate – 42g

Ingredient Spotlight - Almond Milk

Almond milk is basically almonds and water, and is lower in calories than other milks as long as it is unsweetened. Free of cholesterol and saturated fat, and high in healthy fats, it provides a number of important health benefits.

However, you should be aware that commercially produced almond milk is mostly water, sweetener and a thickener, and so should be avoided. It's much better to make your own by soaking one cup of almonds overnight and then blending it with three cups of water. Then remove the pulp with a strainer.

Mango Mash

Mangoes are a delicious fruit to eat at any time of the day but seem particularly suited to breakfast. Add milk and yoghurt to boost the nutrient content, and banana for extra taste and texture.

Ingredients

1 mango
1/2 banana
1/2 cup low-fat milk
1/4 cup low-fat yoghurt

Preparation

Chop the mango and banana into chunks before placing in the blender. Add the milk and yoghurt and blend until smooth.

Nutrition

Calories – 283g
Fibre – 5.5g
Fat – 3g
Protein – 7.5g
Carbohydrate – 60g

Ingredient Spotlight - Mangoes

Mangoes are one of the most beneficial fruits you can eat. They have properties that fight cancer, alkalise the body, aid in weight loss, regulate diabetes and help digestion.

Mangoes are also thought to have aphrodisiac qualities and, in some quarters, are called the 'love fruit'. This is probably because they are extremely rich in vitamin E, which helps to regulate sex hormones and boost sex drive.

Oats Supreme

Add a twist to the traditional oatmeal breakfast by combining it with raspberries, yoghurt and just a touch of ginger.

Ingredients

1/4 cup oats

1/2 cup raspberries

1/2 cup low-fat yoghurt

1 teaspoon honey

1/2 piece of root ginger

1/2 cup water

Preparation

Place the oats and the water in the blender and leave for about 30 minutes. When the oats have softened, add the rest of the ingredients and blend until smooth.

Nutrition

Calories – 155g

Fibre – 6g

Fat – 2.5g

Protein – 5.5g

Carbohydrate – 29g

Ingredient Spotlight - Oats

High in fibre and protein, and low in fat, oats are very good for you. With regard to calories, a cup has just 160.

They also contain a unique fibre called beta-glucan that has beneficial effects on both cholesterol levels and the body's immune system. Regular oat consumption is known to provide protection against heart disease.

On a Date

This is a very simple and easy-to-make smoothie that takes advantage of the many nutrients found in the humble date.

Ingredients

1/2 cup dates

1 banana

1 cup low-fat milk

4 ice cubes

Preparation

Soften the dates by soaking them in the milk for about an hour beforehand. Then add to the blender with the ice and banana and blend until smooth and frothy.

Nutrition

Calories – 465g

Fibre – 11g

Fat – 3g

Protein – 12g

Carbohydrate – 106g

Ingredient Spotlight - Dates

Dates are free from cholesterol and contain a minimal amount of fat. They are rich in vitamins, minerals, protein and fibre. Due to their high content of natural sugars such as glucose, sucrose and fructose, they are also a great energy booster and provide the perfect start to the day.

The significant amount of minerals they contain make dates a superfood for strengthening bones and fighting off debilitating diseases like osteoporosis.

Minty Apple

Full of fruit, the Minty Apple is an extremely tasty smoothie. It contains loads of the fibre and nutrients necessary to kick-start your system.

Ingredients

1 apple
1 pear
1 carrot
1 plum
3/4 cup water
4 mint leaves

Preparation

Place the mint leaves in the blender first and then add the rest of the ingredients. Blend until smooth.

Nutrition

Calories – 236g
Fibre – 12g
Fat – 0.5g
Protein – 2g
Carbohydrate – 61g

Ingredient Spotlight - Apples

Apples are extremely rich in antioxidants, flavanoids and fibre. The phytonutrients and antioxidants help reduce the risk of developing breast cancer, hypertension, diabetes, and heart disease.

Apples can protect against oxidative stress-induced neurotoxicity and may play an important role in reducing the risk of disorders such as Alzheimer's disease.

Papaya Punch

A classic breakfast smoothie that looks as good as it tastes. Not only is it highly nutritious, it is extremely refreshing.

Ingredients

1/2 cup spinach

1/2 cup papaya

1/2 cup watermelon

1/2 pear

1 cup crushed ice

Preparation

Place the spinach in the blender first, then add the other ingredients. Blend until smooth.

Nutrition

Calories – 105g

Fibre – 5g

Fat – 0g

Protein – 1.5g

Carbohydrate – 27g

Ingredient Spotlight - Papayas

Papaya is good for a number of ailments, including heart disease and rheumatoid arthritis. It is rich in fibre, vitamin C and antioxidants that prevent cholesterol building up in the arteries.

Papaya also contains the flavonoid beta-carotene, which helps protect against lung and mouth cancers.

Blue Kiwi

The Blue Kiwi is a delicious smoothie built around three different fruits, and coconut. Too many of these and you'll be on a south sea island before you know it!

Ingredients

1 kiwi
1/2 cup blueberries
1/2 cup pineapple
1/2 cup coconut water
2 or 3 ice cubes

Preparation

Chop the kiwi and the pineapple into chunks. Place in the blender with the rest of the ingredients. Add the ice cubes last and then blend until smooth.

Nutrition

Calories – 147g
Fibre – 5.5g
Fat – 0.5g
Protein – 2.5g
Carbohydrate – 36g

Ingredient Spotlight - Kiwis

Kiwi fruit is high in vitamin C, which boosts the immune system and fights stress and aging. It also promotes iron absorption for healthy bones, blood vessels, and teeth.

These fruits contain a rare, fat-free form of vitamin E that helps lower cholesterol and boost immunity.

Just Fruit

Strawberries and watermelon are both excellent fruits with which to start the day. This energy-packed breakfast smoothie combines them with grapes and guava.

Ingredients

1 guava

1/2 cup grapes

1/2 cup watermelon

1/2 cup strawberries

1/2 cup crushed ice

Preparation

Place all the ingredients in the blender with the ice going in last. Blend until smooth. You can use grapes of any colour.

Nutrition

Calories – 163g

Fibre – 7g

Fat – 1g

Protein – 4g

Carbohydrate – 38g

Ingredient Spotlight - Grapes

Grapes contain powerful antioxidants known as polyphenols that may slow or prevent many types of cancer. These include cancers of the lung, mouth, pharynx, pancreas, prostate and colon.

The resveratrol in red wine, that is well known for being good for the heart, comes from the skins of red grapes.

CHAPTER 4

Smoothies That Keep You Young

While none of us can stop the march of time, it is becoming increasingly apparent that there is a lot we can do to slow it down. Research (not to mention plain common sense) shows that many of the things that have hitherto been accepted as an inevitable consequence of growing old, such as being over-weight, various diseases and illnesses, and mental issues, are actually more to do with the food we eat and the amount of exercise we take.

With regard to food, a diet rich in fruit, vegetables, fish and nuts, will not just keep you looking younger for longer but will also keep you much fitter; both physically and mentally. In this chapter, we look at smoothies that can help in this regard.

Pleasantly Plump

Red peppers, plums and kiwis all contain a large amount of age-defying vitamin C. Together, they create a smoothie that can fight the signs of aging by keeping the skin smooth.

Ingredients

2 kiwis
2 plums
1 red pepper
3/4 cup water

Preparation

Add all the ingredients to the blender and blend until nice and smooth.

Nutrition

Calories – 154g
Fibre – 7g
Fat – 1g
Protein – 4g
Carbohydrate – 38g

Ingredient Spotlight - Plums

Plums help the body to produce and absorb iron, which leads to better blood circulation. This is good for the repair and growth of cell tissue.

Plums are also a natural laxative and are good for relieving constipation. They provide bulk that promotes the movement of faecal matter through the colon, thus helping to prevent colon cancer.

Beetroot Booster

The Beetroot Booster is loaded, not just with vitamin C, but also a wide range of nutrients thanks to the beet content. It is also very high in fibre.

Ingredients

1 beet
1/2 cup blackberries
1/2 cup watermelon
3/4 cup coconut water

Preparation

Add all the ingredients to the blender and blend until nice and smooth.

Nutrition

Calories – 103g
Fibre – 8.5g
Fat – 0.5g
Protein – 4g
Carbohydrate – 26g

Ingredient Spotlight - Beetroots

Beets are high in carbohydrates, which means they are a good and reliable source of energy.

They also contain many nutrients that include sodium, calcium, magnesium, iron and phosphorus. These are all important compounds in the fight against aging.

Studies have shown that beet offers protection against cancer, especially colon cancer.

Watermelon Wine

This age-defying smoothie will delay the formation of unsightly lines and wrinkles in the skin thanks to its high vitamin C and E content. This helps reduce skin damage caused by free radicals.

Ingredients

1/2 cup raspberries

1/2 cup watermelon

1/2 mango

3/4 cup water

Preparation

Add all the ingredients to the blender and blend until nice and smooth.

Nutrition

Calories – 126g

Fibre – 6g

Fat – 1g

Protein – 2g

Carbohydrate – 30g

Ingredient Spotlight - Watermelon

Watermelon is packed with some of the most important antioxidants found in nature. Red watermelon, in particular, is a source of the carotene antioxidant known as lycopene.

These antioxidants travel throughout the body neutralizing the free radicals that can cause so much damage, including to the skin.

Pomegranate Protector

Another smoothie that has excellent skin-protecting properties. All the ingredients provide nutrients that contribute to this.

Ingredients

1/2 pomegranate

1/4 avocado

1 banana

1/2 apple

1 cup water

Preparation

Place all the ingredients in the blender and blend until nice and smooth. Avocado is extremely rich and soft and will give the smoothie a creamy consistency.

Nutrition

Calories – 275g

Fibre – 9g

Fat – 7.5g

Protein – 3g

Carbohydrate – 57g

Ingredient Spotlight - Pomegranates

Pomegranates are a rich source of riboflavin, phosphorus and other vitamins and minerals that promote healthy skin. They do this by increasing its collagen, which is what gives the skin its firmness and elasticity.

Pomegranate is also helpful in lowering the levels of bad cholesterol in the body. Furthermore, it acts as a blood thinner, thus preventing blood clots from forming - blood clots, of course, can cause strokes and heart attacks.

Berry Smooth

This is an absolutely delicious smoothie that is not just refreshing but also loaded with nutrients that feed both the skin and the hair.

Ingredients
1/3 cup blueberries
1/3 cup raspberries
1/3 cup blackberries
1/3 cup strawberries
1/3 cup grapes
3/4 cup crushed ice

Preparation
Simply pile everything into the blender and blend until smooth. Add the ice last otherwise the smoothie may be too watery.

Nutrition
Calories – 139g
Fibre – 7.5g
Fat – 1g
Protein – 2g
Carbohydrate – 29.5g

Ingredient Spotlight - Blackberries
As with most fruits, blackberries are packed with antioxidants, particularly anthocyanocides and polyphenols, that neutralize free radicals and repair the damage caused by the sun. These are both causes of premature aging and skin pigmentation issues.

Blackberries are 85 percent water and so help to keep your skin properly hydrated – this is very important in keeping those wrinkles at bay.

Green Goddess

The Green Goddess is an all-rounder that has anti-aging effects on several parts of the body. Principal to this are the avocado and the spinach, both of which are considered to be superfoods.

Ingredients

1 cup spinach
1 banana
1/4 avocado
1/2 lime
1 tablespoon sunflower seeds
1 cup unsweetened almond milk

Preparation

Blend the sunflower seeds with the almond milk first. Peel the lime and then add with the other ingredients and blend until smooth.

Nutrition

Calories – 300g
Fibre – 9.5g
Fat – 13g
Protein – 6g
Carbohydrate – 37g

Ingredient Spotlight - Avocados

Avocados contain a huge variety of nutrients, including 20 different vitamins and minerals. These include vitamin E and the B-complex vitamins, both of which are very good for your skin.

The potassium they contains helps keep the skin moisturised and hydrated.

Potato Sweetie

Sweet potatoes are packed with vitamin A, which is essential for healthy skin and hair. They contain many other important vitamins and minerals as well.

Ingredients

1 small sweet potato

1 banana

1 tablespoon protein powder

1 cup unsweetened almond milk

1/2 cup water

Preparation

Cook the sweet potato first. Then add to the blender with the other ingredients and blend until smooth.

Nutrition

Calories – 375g

Fibre – 6.5g

Fat – 4.5g

Protein – 25g

Carbohydrate – 58g

Ingredient Spotlight - Sweet Potatoes

This orange-fleshed tubor is prized throughout Africa, India and the Caribbean for the amount of vitamin A and beta-carotene it provides.

Carotenoids are powerful antioxidants that help ward off cancer and protect against the effects of aging. They also help strengthen eyesight and boost immunity to disease.

Young at Heart

This delicious smoothie will hydrate and moisturise your skin, fight free radicals and make you feel younger.

Ingredients
1 cup kale
1/2 cup pineapple
1/2 mango
3/4 cup coconut water

Preparation
Add the ingredients to the blender and blend until smooth. Using frozen pineapple instead of fresh will make the smoothie colder and more refreshing.

Nutrition
Calories – 157g
Fibre – 6g
Fat – 1.5g
Protein – 2.5g
Carbohydrate – 42g

Ingredient Spotlight - Kale

Kale is one of the healthiest and most nutritious plant foods in existence. It helps maintain healthy skin and hair, aids digestion and lowers the risk of heart disease.

Kale is high in vitamin A, a nutrient required for sebum production that keeps hair moisturised, and is necessary for the growth of all body tissues, including skin and hair.

Kale is also high in vitamin C, which the body needs to produce collagen – required to provide structure to skin and hair.

Strawberry Fields

Packed with minerals and phytonutrients, this smoothie gets to parts of the body that others can't reach. The watermelon makes it nice and juicy while the cranberries impart a delicious flavour.

Ingredients

1/2 cup strawberries

1/2 cup cranberries

1/2 cup watermelon

1 banana

3/4 cup coconut water

Preparation

Place all the ingredients in the blender and blend until nice and smooth.

Nutrition

Calories – 194g

Fibre – 7g

Fat – 1g

Protein – 3.5g

Carbohydrate – 50g

Ingredient Spotlight - Strawberries

Strawberries contain a vitamin called biotin, which helps build strong hair and nails. They also contain the antioxidant ellagic acid, which protects the elastic fibres in the skin and helps to prevent sagging.

One cup of strawberries has 136 percent of the recommended daily amount of vitamin C. This helps to ward off wrinkles and age-related dryness of the skin.

CHAPTER 5

Smoothies to Detoxify Your Body

Detoxification (also known as body cleansing) is a procedure that aims to rid the body of 'toxins' – accumulated harmful substances that exert undesirable effects on individual health in the short or long term.

In this chapter, we look at a number of smoothies designed to help you do this. However, you should be aware that for these smoothies to be effective, you need to be taking them (and nothing else) for a minimum of three days. This is the length of time it takes for food (and the toxins) to pass through and out of your body.

Orange & Ginger

Containing ginger, which is excellent for digestion; and orange, which provides a shed-load of vitamins, this sharp-tasting smoothie helps fight off viral infections and purify the blood.

Ingredients

1 banana

1/2 mango

1 small orange

1/2 piece of root ginger

1/2 cup crushed ice

Preparation

Place all the ingredients in the blender and blend until smooth. Put the ice in the blender last.

Nutrition

Calories – 250g

Fibre – 8.5g

Fat – 1g

Protein – 3.5g

Carbohydrate – 60g

Ingredient Spotlight - Ginger

Ginger has been used for centuries to reduce inflammation and treat inflammatory conditions. The phenolic compounds it contains are known to help relieve gastrointestinal irritation, stimulate saliva and bile production, and suppress gastric contractions and movement of food and fluids through the gastrointestinal tract.

All this helps in detoxing your body.

Celery Cleanse

This nutritious smoothie is full of important vitamins and omega-3s essential for ridding the body of environmental toxins, pesticides and harmful minerals.

Ingredients

1 cup kale

1 apple

2 celery sticks

1 tablespoon chia seeds

1 lime

1/4 cup water

Preparation

Blend the chia seeds with the water first. Add the kale next, followed by the other ingredients. Peel the lime. Blend until smooth.

Nutrition

Calories – 213g

Fibre – 11g

Fat – 4.5g

Protein – 4g

Carbohydrate – 45g

Ingredient Spotlight - Celery

Celery aids digestion. Its high water and insoluble fibre content greatly enhances the easy passage of stools.

Celery is also a great internal cleanser and detoxifier for the body. Highly alkalising and hydrating, many of the nutrients in celery are particularly good at cleansing the kidneys.

Hail to Kale

Kale is full of fibre, vitamins and antioxidants, has minimal calories and absolutely no fat. This smoothie is one of the tastiest ways to get some healthy greens down your neck, and help your system clean itself.

Ingredients

1 cup kale

1/4 avocado

1/2 cup cucumber

1/2 lemon

1/2 piece of root ginger

1 cup coconut water

Preparation

Place the kale in the blender first. Peel the lemon. Then add the other ingredients and blend until smooth.

Nutrition

Calories – 190g

Fibre – 8.5g

Fat – 8.5g

Protein – 4.5g

Carbohydrate – 29g

Ingredient Spotlight - Cucumber

Consisting of 95 percent water, cucumbers are naturally low in calories, fat and cholesterol. Their high water content helps the body flush out built-up toxins and also helps keep skin supple and smooth.

Cucumber is well known for its ability to keep blood pressure under control.

Parsley Pride

Containing parsley and avocado, this smoothie provides a twin-barrel attack on those unhealthy and unwanted toxins.

Ingredients

1 cup parsley

1 pear

1/4 avocado

1 tablespoon honey

1 cup water

Preparation

Place the parsley in the blender first. Then add the other ingredients and blend until smooth.

Nutrition

Calories – 260g

Fibre – 10.5g

Fat – 7g

Protein – 3.5g

Carbohydrate – 50g

Ingredient Spotlight - Parsley

Parsley is a nutritional powerhouse with vitamins A, B, C and K, and the minerals iron and potassium. It's a natural diuretic, which helps to eliminate excess fluid without depleting the body of potassium.

Parsley has been shown to suppress over-stimulated immune responses. This makes it a key player in the fight against allergies, and auto-immune and chronic inflammatory disorders.

Pineapple Power

The ingredients in this smoothie not only combine to provide a great taste, they also act to detoxify your body. This is a powerful smoothie that will do you a power of good.

Ingredients

1 cup spinach
1/2 cup pineapple
1/2 apple
2 celery sticks
1/2 lime
1 cup water

Preparation

Put the spinach in the blender first. Then add the other ingredients and blend until smooth.

Nutrition

Calories – 118g
Fibre – 6.5g
Fat – 0g
Protein – 3g
Carbohydrate – 29g

Ingredient Spotlight - Limes

Limes provide a whole range of vital nutrients. These include antioxidants, flavonol glycosides, kaempferol and vitamin C. These all help to stave off colds and flu, and ease arthritis pain.

They may also help prevent many diseases, such as heart disease, stroke hardening of the arteries, and cancers of the skin, stomach, lung, breast, colon and mouth.

The Kiwi

Beets are packed with toxin-flushing vitamins and minerals, including magnesium, zinc, iron, and calcium. When paired with digestion-friendly carrot, the result is a great body detoxifier.

Ingredients

1 carrot
1 beet
1 tomato
1 kiwi
3/4 cup water

Preparation

Place all the ingredients in the blender and blend until nice and smooth.

Nutrition

Calories – 124g
Fibre – 7.5g
Fat – 0.5g
Protein – 3g
Carbohydrate – 29g

Ingredient Spotlight - Carrots

Carrots contain oils that work on the mucus membranes of the stomach and colon. This helps with digestion and gets the bowels functioning properly. Stool size and softness increases making them easier to pass.

This all helps in the process of detoxification.

The Green Detoxifier

The Green Detoxifier is a toxin-defying mix of greens, fruit, seeds and yoghurt that is not only full of vitamins for boundless energy but also body-cleansing fibre.

Ingredients

1 cup broccoli

1/4 avocado

1/2 banana

1/2 orange

1 tablespoon chia seeds

1/2 cup low-fat yoghurt

1 cup water

Preparation

Blend the chia seeds with the water first. Then add the broccoli and the other ingredients. Blend again until smooth.

Nutrition

Calories – 298g

Fibre – 12.5g

Fat – 11.5g

Protein – 10g

Carbohydrate – 46g

Ingredient Spotlight - Chia Seeds

Despite their small size, chia seeds are packed full of important nutrients. They are an excellent source of omega-3 fatty acids, which help to raise HDL cholesterol (the good cholesterol). They also contain a lot of fibre, which prevents constipation and promotes regularity for a healthy digestive tract.

Cabbage Cocktail

'Cabbage Cocktail' may not sound too appetizing but rest assured, your body will love it. Cabbage is well known for its ability to clear out your digestive system.

Ingredients

1 cup cabbage

1 carrot

1 tomato

1/2 pepper

3/4 cup water

Preparation

Put the cabbage in the blender first, add the other ingredients and blend until smooth.

Nutrition

Calories – 84g

Fibre – 6g

Fat – 0g

Protein – 3g

Carbohydrate – 20g

Ingredient Spotlight - Cabbage

The fibre and water content in cabbage help prevent constipation, thus promoting a healthy digestive tract. Eating an adequate amount of fibre promotes regularity, which is crucial for the daily excretion of toxins.

The pepper and carrot in this smoothie further add to its ability to detoxify your body.

Cherries & Berries

The berries in this smoothie activate detoxifying enzymes in the body while the ginger stimulates the digestive system. Plus, it tastes just great.

Ingredients
1/2 cup grapefruit
1/2 cup blueberries
1/2 cup cherries
1/2 inch piece of root ginger
1 teaspoon honey
3/4 cup unsweetened almond milk

Preparation
Place all the ingredients in the blender and blend until nice and smooth.

Nutrition
Calories – 194g
Fibre – 5.5g
Fat – 2.5g
Protein – 2.5g
Carbohydrate – 42g

Ingredient Spotlight - Cherries
Cherries are a rich source of vitamins, minerals and antioxidants, which aid in digestion, reduce inflammation and help rid the body of free radicals.

Cherries also contain pectin, which helps to remove heavy metals, synthetic chemicals used as food additives, cholesterol and other toxins in the intestines.

CHAPTER 6

Smoothies To Boost Brain Power

The brain is an energy-hungry organ. Despite comprising only two percent of the body's weight, it uses more than 20 percent of daily energy intake. Because of this, the foods we consume greatly affect brain function, including learning, memory, emotions, cognition, etc.

Unfortunately, the typical westerner eats too much of the wrong kinds of food and not enough of the right kinds. So, our brains do not get the energy we need even though we eat plenty overall.

One simple solution to this is the smoothie. Quick to prepare and consume, a smoothie enables you to give your brain all the nutrients it needs. Foods rich in omega-3 fatty acids, the B family of vitamins, and vitamins C, D, and E are the ones to go for.

Coconut Cream

This banana, coconut and apple concoction contains a number of essential nutrients for the brain. That apart, you will also find that it is a very pleasant drink in its own right.

Ingredients

1 banana

1 apple

3 tablespoons of coconut meat

1/2 cup unsweetened almond milk

1/2 cup crushed ice

Preparation

Place all the ingredients in the blender and blend until smooth. Put the ice in last.

Nutrition

Calories – 380g

Fibre – 11g

Fat – 15g

Protein – 4g

Carbohydrate – 64g

Ingredient Spotlight - Coconuts

Coconut contains low amounts of natural sugars and high amounts of fibre and manganese. It also happens to be nature's richest source of medium-chain triglycerides.

Medium-chain triglycerides are converted into a stable source of fuel for your brain and have been found to boost cognitive performance in adults suffering from memory disorders such as Alzheimer's disease.

Mango Mayhem

The Mango Mayhem is a delightfully flavoured smoothie that also packs a range of omega-3 fatty acids, beta-carotene and other brain-boosting compounds that you simply cannot do without.

Ingredients

1 mango

1 tomato

1 kiwi

1 tablespoon pumpkin seeds

3/4 cup unsweetened almond milk

2 or 3 ice cubes

Preparation

Blend the pumpkin seeds with the almond milk first. Then add the other ingredients and blend until smooth.

Nutrition

Calories – 310g

Fibre – 8g

Fat – 7.5g

Protein – 6.5g

Carbohydrate – 57g

Ingredient Spotlight - Pumpkin Seeds

Pumpkin seeds are nutritional powerhouses and contain a wide variety of nutrients ranging from magnesium and manganese to copper, protein and zinc.

They are also one of the best sources of plant-based omega-3s, which play an important role in cognitive function.

Just Berries

As refreshing as it is nutritious, this delicious smoothie will ensure your brain is in top gear and stays that way. The blueberries are the key ingredient in this one.

Ingredients

1 cup blueberries

1/2 cup raspberries

2 tablespoons raisins

1/2 lemon

3/4 cup crushed ice

Preparation

Peel the lemon and then place all the ingredients in the blender with the ice going in last. Blend until smooth.

Nutrition

Calories – 177g

Fibre – 12.5g

Fat – 1g

Protein – 2.5g

Carbohydrate – 45g

Ingredient Spotlight - Blueberries

Blueberries have been called 'brainberries' and have just about the highest antioxidant capacity of all the many fruits and vegetables. They protect the brain from oxidative stress, and can reduce the effects of age-related conditions such as Alzheimer's disease and dementia.

Furthermore, the antioxidants can improve memory and other brain functions.

Avocado Special

All the ingredients in this powerful smoothie are known to have brain-enhancing properties – the avocado in particular. Get your thinking cap on now and blend one up!

Ingredients
1/2 avocado
1/4 cup broccoli
1/4 cucumber
1/4 pepper
1 garlic clove
3 sage leaves
1 1/2 cups water

Preparation
Place the sage leaves and broccoli in the blender first. Then add the other ingredients and blend until smooth.

Nutrition
Calories – 170g
Fibre – 7.5g
Fat – 13.5g
Protein – 3g
Carbohydrate – 13.5g

Ingredient Spotlight - Avocados
Avocados are almost as good as blueberries at promoting brain health. They are rich in mono-unsaturated fat, which contributes to healthy blood flow in the brain.

They also help to lower blood pressure, which can reduce the risks of hypertension or stroke that can permanently damage brain tissue.

Chia & Blueberry

The Chia & Blueberry is a deliciously fruity smoothie that combines the nutritional punch of the berries and banana with the omega-3-rich chia seeds.

Ingredients

1/2 cup blueberries

1/2 cup raspberries

1/2 cup cranberries

1 banana

1 tablespoon chia seeds

1 cup water

Preparation

Blend the chia seeds with the water first. Then add the rest of the ingredients and blend again until smooth.

Nutrition

Calories – 258g

Fibre – 13g

Fat – 4g

Protein – 4.5g

Carbohydrate – 55g

Ingredient Spotlight - Bananas

Bananas are high in vitamin B6, which is crucial to efficient brain function.

Another vital nutrient in banana is magnesium. Magnesium helps the body excrete ammonia - this can inhibit focus and reduce attention span. It also assists in electrical activities between brain nerve cells.

Egg Head

This smoothie packs a considerable punch thanks to its high protein content. The eggplant (also known as aubergine) will have your brain cells buzzing.

Ingredients

1 cup eggplant

1 banana

1/2 teaspoon cinnamon

1 tablespoon whey protein powder

3/4 cup soya milk

Preparation

Place all the ingredients in the blender, apart from the protein powder. Blend until smooth and then add the protein powder. Blend again.

Nutrition

Calories – 279g

Fibre – 7g

Fat – 5g

Protein – 32g

Carbohydrate – 45g

Ingredient Spotlight - Eggplants

Eggplants are wonderful sources of phytonutrients, which boost cognitive activity and general mental health.

They not only defend against free radical activity and keep your body and brain safe from toxins and diseases, they also increase blood flow to the brain. This boosts the powers of memory and analytic thought.

Pomegranate Promise

Fibre helps regulate the blood's glucose (sugar), which is the brain's main source of energy. This smoothie is full of fibre, along with other brain-friendly antioxidants.

Ingredients
1 pomegranate
1/2 cup strawberries
1 tablespoon honey
1/2 cup low-fat yoghurt

Preparation
Blend the pomegranate seeds with the yoghurt first. Then add the strawberries and honey and blend until smooth.

Nutrition
Calories – 257g
Fibre – 3g
Fat – 2g
Protein – 5g
Carbohydrate – 57g

Ingredient Spotlight - Pomegranates

Regular consumption of pomegranate has a lot of health benefits. These include the prevention of neuro-inflammation related to memory loss and Alzheimer's disease.

Pomegranate is a highly-concentrated source of antioxidants and this is the key to the fruit's neuro-protective properties.

Blue Beetle

Beets are high in fibre, phytonutrients, folate, beta-carotene and natural nitrates that increase blood flow to the brain. These all contribute to overall brain health.

Ingredients

1/2 cup blueberries
1/2 beet
1 carrot
1/2 lime
1/2 inch piece of root ginger
3/4 cup unsweetened almond milk

Preparation

Peel the lime before placing in the blender. Add the rest of the ingredients and blend until smooth.

Nutrition

Calories – 156g
Fibre – 5.5g
Fat – 1g
Protein – 3.5g
Carbohydrate – 35g

Ingredient Spotlight - Beets

Beets are high in vitamin C, fibre, and essential minerals. These include potassium which is important for healthy nerve and muscle function; and manganese which is good for bones, liver, kidneys, and the pancreas.

Eating beets increases blood flow to the brain and so can help fight the progression of dementia.

Green Heaven

A robust mix of both fruits and vegetables, the Green Heaven will keep your mind active and alert.

Ingredients
1/2 cup cantaloupe
1/2 cup kale
1/2 cup spinach
1/2 apple
1/2 banana
1 cup water

Preparation
Put the kale and spinach in the blender first. Then add the other ingredients and blend until smooth.

Nutrition
Calories – 141
Fibre – 5g
Fat – 1g
Protein – 2.5g
Carbohydrate – 35g

Ingredient Spotlight - Cantaloupes

A member of the melon family, cantaloupe has an abundant supply of potassium - a mineral that relaxes the blood vessels and reduces blood pressure.

Potassium also increases the flow of blood and oxygen to the brain, which helps it function more efficiently.

CHAPTER 7

Smoothies For The Digestive System

For people with digestive disorders or inflammatory bowel diseases, the consumption of digestion-friendly smoothies is highly recommended. Made with suitable ingredients, they can improve the absorption of nutrients and the general health of the digestive system considerably.

Smoothies contain the two most important elements for good digestive health – water and fibre. This makes them the perfect solution to digestive issues because they enable the body to get the vitamins and minerals it needs in an assimilable form that doesn't overtax the digestive system.

Watermelon Wonder

The Watermelon Wonder is an extremely nourishing smoothie that contains watermelon, tomato, banana and hemp seeds. It is particularly good for the digestive system.

Ingredients

1 cup watermelon

1 tomato

1 banana

1 tablespoon hemp seeds

3/4 cup water

Preparation

Blend the hemp seeds with the water first. Then add the rest of the ingredients and blend again until smooth.

Nutrition

Calories – 256g

Fibre – 5.5g

Fat – 2g

Protein – 8.5g

Carbohydrate – 44g

Ingredient Spotlight - Hemp Seeds

Fibre is an essential part of a healthy diet and is linked with better digestive health. Hemp seeds are a great source of both soluble and insoluble fibre.

The former is a valuable source of nutrients while the latter adds bulk to faecal matter and helps food and waste pass through the intestines.

Coconut Cooler

This digestion-friendly smoothie is as refreshing as it is healthy. Those watching their waistline should beware the calories added by the coconut, though.

Ingredients

1 cup pineapple

1 banana

1/2 cup coconut meat

1 tablespoon fennel seeds

3/4 cup water

Preparation

Blend the fennel seeds with the water first. Then add the rest of the ingredients and blend again until smooth.

Nutrition

Calories – 357g

Fibre – 12g

Fat – 14g

Protein – 5g

Carbohydrate – 61g

Ingredient Spotlight - Fennel Seeds

Fennel is highly beneficial in relieving digestive problems such as indigestion, bloating, flatulence, constipation, intestinal gas and irritable bowels.

Fresh fennel works as a natural fat buster by boosting the metabolism and breaking down fats. Plus, being a diuretic, fennel helps reduce water retention, which is a common cause of temporary weight gain.

Appletizer

A fruit smoothie that incorporates a surprising amount of that all-important fibre for good digestive health.

Ingredients

1 apple

1/2 avocado

1/2 cup blueberries

1 cup water

Preparation

Place the ingredients in the blender and blend until nice and smooth.

Nutrition

Calories – 282g

Fibre – 12g

Fat – 14g

Protein – 3g

Carbohydrate – 43g

Ingredient Spotlight - Apples

Apples contain insoluble fibre, particularly the skin. This type of fibre provides bulk in the intestinal tract and helps hold water, soften the stools and move food quickly through the intestines.

It also helps to reduce the risk of diverticular disease, which causes abdominal pain, changes in bowel habits, cramping, vomiting and nausea. This can lead to complications such as infections, bleeding, small tears and blockages in the colon.

Yummy Yoghurt

The Yummy Yoghurt is another fibre-packed smoothie that will keep your digestive system in good working order. The raspberries alone have nearly 25 percent of your daily fibre requirement.

Ingredients

1/2 cup papaya
1/2 cup raspberries
1/4 cup Greek yoghurt
1/2 cup water

Preparation

Place the ingredients in the blender and blend until nice and smooth.

Nutrition

Calories – 92g
Fibre – 5g
Fat – 2g
Protein – 4.5g
Carbohydrate – 26g

Ingredient Spotlight - Yoghurt

Greek yoghurt has a high content of micro-organisms called probiotics. These help to stop bad or undesirable bacteria from growing in the gastrointestinal tract, thus preventing diarrhoea, irritable bowel syndrome and colon diseases.

Vitamin B12 is essential for energy and healthy brain function. Vegetarians are often deficient in B12 because it is found mainly in meat. Greek yoghurt is full of it and so is an excellent meat-free way to add more to the diet.

The Ginger Kiwi

Quick to make, the Ginger Kiwi smoothie is an excellent aid to good digestion. It tastes good as well.

Ingredients

2 kiwis

1/2 cucumber

2 celery sticks

1/2 inch piece of root ginger

3/4 cup unsweetened almond milk

Preparation

Place all the ingredients in the blender and blend until nice and smooth.

Nutrition

Calories – 159g

Fibre – 6g

Fat – 3g

Protein – 4g

Carbohydrate – 31g

Ingredient Spotlight - Kiwis

Kiwis are excellent for the digestive system in several ways. They aid the digestion of protein, which could otherwise lead to a build-up of toxins in the large intestine.

They also relieve constipation and help to produce bulkier and softer stools, as well as more frequent stool production. Yet another benefit is that they improve bowel function for people who suffer from irritable bowel syndrome.

Broccoli Blaster

This is a well-named smoothie that will quite literally blast your digestive system clear of all unwanted substances. Actually, this may be somewhat of an exaggeration but you get the picture!

Ingredients

1 cup broccoli
1 cup spinach
4 prunes
3 or 4 mint leaves
3/4 cup water

Preparation

Place the broccoli, spinach and mint leaves in the blender first. Then add the prunes and water and blend until smooth.

Nutrition

Calories – 123g
Fibre – 6g
Fat – 0g
Protein – 3.5g
Carbohydrate – 28g

Ingredient Spotlight - Mint

Mint is widely used as a digestive aid. It relaxes the muscular lining of the digestive tract, which relieves cramps and gas, and alleviates indigestion.

It can also significantly reduce abdominal pain and improve quality of life for people with irritable bowel syndrome.

Burdock & Plum

All the ingredients in this pearler of a smoothie are full of fibre. However, the pineapple has another string to its bow – it contains an enzyme called bromelain that helps in breaking down and absorbing protein. This is a great aid to digestion.

Ingredients

1/2 cup pineapple
1/2 cup mango
2 plums
1 inch piece burdock root
3/4 cup crushed ice

Preparation

Place all the ingredients in the blender and blend until nice and smooth.

Nutrition

Calories – 239g
Fibre – 8g
Fat – 0.5g
Protein – 2.5g
Carbohydrate – 59g

Ingredient Spotlight - Burdock Root

Burdock root stimulates digestion by increasing intestinal secretions and digestive acid, so it isn't recommended if you suffer from excess stomach acid, or have ulcers or an irritable bowel.

It also contains prebiotics, which stimulate the growth of healthy bacteria in the gut.

Cranberry Cleaner

Quick and easy to prepare, the Cranberry Cleaner is as delicious as it is healthy. Both cranberries and ginger have well known digestion-friendly properties. The raspberries are excellent as well.

Ingredients

1 cup cranberries

1/2 cup raspberries

1/2 cucumber

1/2 inch piece root ginger

3/4 cup water

Preparation

Place all the ingredients in the blender and blend until nice and smooth.

Nutrition

Calories – 122g

Fibre – 9g

Fat – 1g

Protein – 2g

Carbohydrate – 24g

Ingredient Spotlight - Cranberries

Cranberries contain enzymes that help maintain regular digestive function. They also have anti-inflammatory benefits, which reduce the risk of chronic inflammation in the stomach and large intestine.

Zucchini Zinger

All the ingredients in this smoothie have loads of fibre that work to keep the digestive system in good shape.

Ingredients
1 cup kale
1 carrot
1/2 zucchini (courgette)
1/2 apple
3/4 cup water

Preparation
Place the kale in the blender first and then add the rest of the ingredients. Blend until smooth.

Nutrition
Calories – 126g
Fibre – 6g
Fat – 1.5g
Protein – 3g
Carbohydrate – 28g

Ingredient Spotlight - Zucchinis
Zucchini's dark skin is high in soluble fibre, which slows digestion and stabilises blood sugar levels. This type of fibre can also prevent constipation and relieve irritable bowel symptoms.

Zucchini is high in the heart-healthy mineral potassium. One cup gives you more than 15 percent of the recommended daily amount.

CHAPTER 8

Smoothies That Keep Your Heart Healthy

Most people are aware that in order to keep their heart and arteries in good shape, it is necessary to watch the salt and saturated fat, and eat plenty of fibre.

Smoothies provide a way to do this. When prepared with the right ingredients and enjoyed in moderation, they can provide everything your heart needs including fibre, omega-3 fatty acids and antioxidants.

Raspberry & Walnut

Although it has quite a high sugar content, the Raspberry & Walnut smoothie contains many of the nutrients essential for a healthy heart.

Ingredients

1 beet
1/2 cup brussels sprouts
1/2 cup raspberries
1/4 cup walnuts
3/4 cup unsweetened almond milk

Preparation

Blend the walnuts with the almond milk first. Then add the beet, raspberries and the sprouts and blend again until smooth.

Nutrition

Calories – 331g
Fibre – 10.5g
Fat – 22g
Protein – 9g
Carbohydrate – 30g

Ingredient Spotlight - Raspberries

Raspberries have a high content of polyphenols – antioxidants that eradicate damage-causing free radicals in the body.

They also provide a lot of fibre and vitamin C, both of which limit the risk of stroke. 100g of raspberries provides about 45 percent of the daily amount of vitamin C we require.

Lemon Surprise

Never mind the blues, this incredibly healthy smoothie will lift your heart and have it singing with joy.

Ingredients

1/2 cup broccoli

1/2 cup red grapes

1/4 cup avocado

1/2 lemon

1 tablespoon whey protein powder

1 cup water

Preparation

Place the broccoli in the blender first. Peel the lemon and add it with the rest of the ingredients and blend until smooth.

Nutrition

Calories – 269g

Fibre – 5.5g

Fat – 8g

Protein – 26g

Carbohydrate – 25g

Ingredient Spotlight - Lemons

Lemons are good for the heart due to the fact that they are packed with vitamin C, which helps to maintain healthy cholesterol levels.

High cholesterol is one of the main risk factors with regard to problems of the heart and circulatory system.

Just Strawberries

No artery-clogging cream in this one. Just healthy ingredients that will keep your heart in good shape. The strawberries are extremely beneficial in this respect.

Ingredients

1/2 cup cauliflower

1/2 cup asparagus

1/2 cup strawberries

1 tablespoon chia seeds

3/4 cup water

Preparation

Blend the chia seeds with the water first. Then add the cauliflower, asparagus and strawberries and blend again until smooth.

Nutrition

Calories – 101g

Fibre – 8g

Fat – 3g

Protein – 4.5g

Carbohydrate – 15g

Ingredient Spotlight - Strawberries

Strawberries are rich in a class of flavonoids known as anthocyanins. These are antioxidants that give this fruit its characteristic red colour. Not only do they help prevent the build-up of plaque in the arteries, they also help to keep blood pressure at a healthy level.

Berry Blue

The Berry Blue smoothie contains hemp seeds, which are incredibly rich in omega-3 and omega 6 fatty acids. Almonds add more protein while the blueberries and kale contribute a wide range of important nutrients.

Ingredients

1/2 cup kale
1/2 cup blueberries
1/4 cup almonds
1 tablespoon hemp seeds
1 cup green tea

Preparation

Blend the almonds and hemp seeds with the green tea first. Then add the kale and blueberries and blend again until smooth.

Nutrition

Calories – 322g
Fibre – 7g
Fat – 21g
Protein – 12g
Carbohydrate – 23g

Ingredient Spotlight - Hemp Seeds

The omega-3 fatty acids in hemp seeds reduces the risk of cardiovascular disease, lowers blood pressure, and may even ward off Alzheimer's disease. Hemp seeds are one of the few plant-based sources of omega-3.

The Cholesterol Buster

This smoothie is named The Cholesterol Buster with good reason. Apple and spinach are both high in phytonutrients that provide protection against cholesterol.

Ingredients

1 cup spinach

1 apple

1 tablespoon almond butter

1 clove garlic

3/4 cup soya milk

Preparation

Put the spinach in the blender first. Then add the rest of the ingredients and blend until smooth.

Nutrition

Calories – 304g

Fibre – 7g

Fat – 12.5g

Protein – 11g

Carbohydrate – 41g

Ingredient Spotlight - Spinach

A pigment called lutein found in spinach reduces the risk of heart attacks and strokes by reducing the cholesterol and other fat deposits in the blood vessels.

The Smart Heart

Packed with heart-healthy ingredients, this smoothie not only keeps your cardiovascular system in good order, it is delicious to drink as well.

Ingredients

1 banana

1/2 cup raspberries

1/2 orange

1 teaspoon dark cacao powder (at least 70 percent cacao)

1 tablespoon almond or peanut butter

1/4 cup Greek yoghurt

3/4 cup low-fat milk

Preparation

Place all the ingredients in the blender and blend until nice and smooth.

Nutrition

Calories – 334g

Fibre – 11g

Fat – 13g

Protein – 14.5g

Carbohydrate – 61g

Ingredient Spotlight - Cacao Powder

Dark chocolate can play an important role in protecting against heart disease. It does this by reducing the amount of cholesterol in the arteries, and so lessening the chances of heart attacks and strokes.

Dark chocolate can also reduce insulin resistance, which is another common risk factor for diseases such as heart disease and diabetes.

Tick Tock

This incredibly powerful smoothie will keep your ticker tick-tocking merrily away. The oatmeal makes it thick and creamy thus keeping you feeling full for longer.

Ingredients

1 banana
1/2 cup red grapes
1/4 cup oatmeal
1/4 cup almonds
1 teaspoon honey
1 1/2 cups water

Preparation

Blend the almonds with the water first. Then add the rest of the ingredients and blend until smooth.

Nutrition

Calories – 485g
Fibre – 8.5g
Fat – 21g
Protein – 9.5g
Carbohydrate – 77g

Ingredient Spotlight - Red Grapes

Grapes are rich in two heart-healthy antioxidants called flavonoids and resveratrol. Dark red and purple grapes contain more.

These antioxidants are good for the heart in several ways. They reduce the risk of blood clots, reduce low-density lipoprotein cholesterol, prevent damage to blood vessels in the heart, and keep blood pressure normal.

Walnut Whirl

Nuts of all types are nutrient powerhouses. With regard to the heart, walnuts are the ones to go for due to, amongst other things, their high content of omega-3 fatty acids.

Ingredients

1/2 cup blueberries

1/2 cup pomegranate

1/4 cup avocado

1/4 cup walnuts

4 dates

1 cup coconut water

Preparation

Blend the walnuts with the coconut water first. Then add the rest of the ingredients and blend again until smooth. Alternatively, chop the walnuts finely and sprinkle on top of the smoothie.

Nutrition

Calories – 539g

Fibre – 11g

Fat – 28g

Protein – 9.5g

Carbohydrate – 76g

Ingredient Spotlight - Walnuts

Walnuts contain the omega-3 fat alpha-linolenic acid (ALA), which is anti-inflammatory and can prevent the formation of blood clots. People who have a diet high in ALA are significantly less likely to have a heart attack.

The Happy Heart

The Happy Heart is another heart-friendly smoothie packed with those essential omega-3 fatty acids. This time it's the flax seeds that are the source.

Ingredients

1/2 cup spinach

1/2 cup pineapple

1/2 orange

1/2 banana

1 tablespoon flax seeds

1 cup unsweetened almond milk

Preparation

Blend the flax seeds with the almond milk first. Then add the rest of the ingredients and blend again until smooth.

Nutrition

Calories – 235g

Fibre – 7.5g

Fat – 6g

Protein – 5g

Carbohydrate – 43g

Ingredient Spotlight - Flax seeds

Flax seeds (also called linseeds) are a rich source of micro-nutrients, fibre, manganese, vitamin B1 and the very important omega-3 fatty acid.

The seeds also contain lignans that can reduce cholesterol as well as blood pressure, thus lowering the risk of cardiovascular disease.

CHAPTER 9

Smoothies For the Immune System

Your immune system comprises special cells, proteins, tissues and organs that defend you against germs and micro-organisms every single moment of every single day. In most cases, it does a great job of keeping you healthy and free of infection. But sometimes problems with the immune system can lead to illness.

These problems can be exacerbated by the type of food you eat. So, to keep your immune system healthy, you must restrict your intake of red meat, sugary drinks and snacks, and processed foods. In this chapter, we look at smoothies that include the foods necessary for a strong immune system.

Spicy Banana

The Spicy Banana is not just brilliant for your immune system but for other parts of your body as well.

Ingredients

1 banana
1/2 cup pumpkin
2 celery sticks
1/2 inch piece of root ginger
1 teaspoon of cinnamon
1 cup coconut water

Preparation

Place all the ingredients in the blender and blend until nice and smooth.

Nutrition

Calories – 187g
Fibre – 9g
Fat – 1g
Protein – 4.5g
Carbohydrate – 43g

Ingredient Spotlight - Cinnamon

Cinnamon is known to boost the immune system and helps to ward off colds and flu thanks to its anti-bacterial and anti-microbial properties, and antioxidant activities.

Cinammon can also help the digestive system and prevent bowel movement disorders.

Watermelon & Mint

Watermelon and mint combine well in a smoothie that helps protect you from degenerative diseases, and helps your cells function more efficiently.

Ingredients

1/2 cup watermelon

1/2 cup papaya

1 banana

4 or five mint leaves

3/4 cup water

Preparation

Put the mint in the blender first. Then add the rest of the ingredients and blend until smooth.

Nutrition

Calories – 157g

Fibre – 4.5g

Fat – 1g

Protein – 1.5g

Carbohydrate – 41g

Ingredient Spotlight - Mint

Mint is full of vitamins and immune system-friendly minerals like vitamin A, C, calcium, iron, potassium, magnesium and phosphorous. These give the immune system a considerable boost.

Red & Blue

The main ingredient in this one is red cabbage, a vegetable known to provide immune system benefits. Toss in some blueberries and you have a great immune system-friendly smoothie.

Ingredients

1 cup red cabbage

1/2 cup blueberries

1/2 cucumber

1 tangerine

3/4 cup water

Preparation

Put the cabbage in the blender first. Then add the rest of the ingredients and blend until smooth.

Nutrition

Calories – 101g

Fibre – 6.5g

Fat – 0.5g

Protein – 2.5g

Carbohydrate – 28g

Ingredient Spotlight - Red Cabbage

Red cabbage is an excellent source of important antioxidants that not only boost the immune system in general but also it's ability to fight cancer.

These antioxidants include polyphenols that also protect the body against free radicals and aging.

Taste of the Tropics

Pineapple, mango and kale are all very rich in vitamin C. Pineapple also contains vitamin B6. These vitamins are essential for proper functioning of the immune system.

Ingredients

1/2 cup pineapple
1/2 cup mango
1/2 cup kale
1/2 lime
3/4 cup coconut water

Preparation

Put the kale in the blender first. Peel the lime and add it with the rest of the ingredients and blend until smooth.

Nutrition

Calories – 187g
Fibre – 7g
Fat – 1.5g
Protein – 2.5g
Carbohydrate – 42g

Ingredient Spotlight - Pineapples

Pineapple has more than 130 percent of our daily requirement of vitamin C. This vitamin boosts the immune system by stimulating the activity of white blood cells, and by acting as an antioxidant to defend against the harmful effects of free radicals.

In the Limelight

Loaded with vitamin C and anti-inflamatory compounds, the In the the Limelight smoothie is just what you need to keep your body healthy free of disease.

Ingredients

1 cup strawberries

1/2 cup red cabbage

1/2 lime

1 teaspoon maple syrup

3/4 cup almond milk

Preparation

Put the cabbage in the blender first. Peel the lime and add it with the rest of the ingredients and blend until smooth.

Nutrition

Calories – 128g

Fibre – 5g

Fat – 2g

Protein – 2g

Carbohydrate – 29g

Ingredient Spotlight - Limes

Limes contain powerful anti-viral properties and can help to speed up the body's natural healing process.

Consisting of 90 percent water, they are fat-free, and, when they are peeled rather than juiced, provide a large amount of fibre.

Guava Goody

This smoothie is an ideal pick-me-up if you are recovering from illness or are taking antibiotics. It will help get your system back on track.

Ingredients

1 guava
1 kiwi
1/2 cup cherries
1 tablespoon chia seeds
3/4 cup coconut water

Preparation

Blend the chia seeds with the coconut water first. Then add the rest of the ingredients and blend again until smooth.

Nutrition

Calories – 225g
Fibre – 14g
Fat – 5g
Protein – 6.5g
Carbohydrate – 43g

Ingredient Spotlight - Guavas

Along with pineapples, guavas are one of the richest sources of vitamin C, containing four times the amount found in oranges. The fruit should be eaten with the skin as this contains even more.

Guava is also very high in fibre, which makes it an excellent food for the digestive system.

Carrot & Citrus Combo

The ingredients in this power-packed smoothie will have your immune system working overtime.

Ingredients

1 carrot

1 orange

1 tomato

1/2 lemon

3/4 cup water

Preparation

Place all the ingredients in the blender and blend until nice and smooth.

Nutrition

Calories – 118g

Fibre – 6.5g

Fat – 0g

Protein – 3g

Carbohydrate – 28g

Ingredient Spotlight - Carrots

The immune system encompasses several parts of the body that include the lymph nodes, the spleen, white blood cells, the skin and mucosal membranes of the respiratory tract.

The vitamins and minerals abundant in carrots are essential for it to work properly. Carrots contain beta-carotene, which is a powerful phytonutrient that boosts the immune system's production of infection-fighting cells.

Elderberry Honey

The elderberries are the key to this delicious smoothie. They are not just good for your immune system, they are good for your *entire* system.

Ingredients
1/2 cup spinach
1/2 cup elderberries
1 pear
3/4 cup water

Preparation
Place all the ingredients in the blender and blend until smooth. If fresh elderberries are not available, use elderberry extract instead.

Nutrition
Calories – 152g
Fibre – 10.5g
Fat – 0g
Protein – 1.5g
Carbohydrate – 40g

Ingredient Spotlight - Elderberries
Elderberries contain an array of potent anti-viral compounds as well as high amounts of bioflavonoids, Amongst other things, these help fight off colds and flu.

They also provide protection against yeast infections, nasal and chest congestion and hay fever.

Just Peachy

The Just Peachy is an excellent body-protective smoothie that's packed with immune boosters and anti-inflammatory properties. This is due in no small part to the presence of turmeric.

Ingredients

1 peach

1/2 mango

2 figs

1 teaspoon of ground turmeric

3/4 cup water

Preparation

Place all the ingredients in the blender and blend until nice and smooth.

Nutrition

Calories – 192g

Fibre – 7g

Fat – 1g

Protein – 2.5g

Carbohydrate – 47g

Ingredient Spotlight - Peaches

Peaches are rich in ascorbic acid and zinc, both of which help the body to function normally and maintain a healthy immune system.

Zinc and vitamin C contribute to effective wound healing, plus they have antioxidant properties that help in fighting infections and reduce the severity of illnesses such as colds, pneumonia and diarrhoea.

CHAPTER 10

Smoothies For Diabetics

If you're diabetic, you won't need to be told that you must avoid foods that have a high sugar content.

Smoothies built around green vegetables and low-sugar fruits are, however, a different matter. Not only are they an ideal way to get more fruit and vegetables, they can also help reverse some of the diet and lifestyle problems that exacerbate diabetes, or contribute to its progression.

In this chapter, we look at a range of smoothies that are purpose-built for people with diabetes.

Blue Cherry

Containing low-glycemic fruit, the Blue Cherry smoothie is the perfect low-fat, low-calorie, low-carb drink.

Ingredients
1/2 cup cherries
1/2 cup blueberries
1 banana
1/2 lime
3/4 cup water

Preparation
Place the ingredients in the blender and blend until smooth and creamy.

Nutrition
Calories – 194g
Fibre – 5.5g
Fat – 0.5g
Protein – 2g
Carbohydrate – 50g

Ingredient Spotlight - Cherries

Cherries are a low-GI choice and a good addition to a diabetes-friendly diet. They contain compounds called anthocyanins that boost insulin, thus helping to control blood sugar levels.

Cherries are also packed with antioxidants, which can help fight heart disease, cancer, and other diseases.

Mango Tea

Green tea is just about the healthiest thing you can drink. Adding ginger and mango creates a low calorie smoothie with a tropical flavour.

Ingredients

1 carrot

1 mango

1 tomato

1/2 inch piece of root ginger

1 cup green tea

Preparation

Make the green tea first and add to the blender. Add the rest of the ingredients and blend until smooth.

Nutrition

Calories – 195g

Fibre – 8g

Fat – 0.5g

Protein – 2.5g

Carbohydrate – 47g

Ingredient Spotlight - Green Tea

Green tea is not just great for overall health, it can help to target diabetes specifically. It does this by improving insulin sensitivity and so reducing blood sugar levels.

Green tea also slows down the rate of digestion, which means that your body will absorb starches more slowly.

Berry Nice

Containing three different types of antioxidant-rich berries, plus highly nutritious kale, this is a supercharged smoothie ideal for diabetics.

Ingredients

1/2 cup raspberries
1/2 cup blueberries
1/2 cup strawberries
1/2 cup kale
1 cup water

Preparation

Place the kale in the blender first followed by the other ingredients and blend until smooth.

Nutrition

Calories – 115g
Fibre – 8g
Fat – 1.5g
Protein – 2g
Carbohydrate – 29g

Ingredient Spotlight - Kale

Rich in nutrients such as magnesium and vitamin K, kale helps to control blood sugar. This is due to it's high fibre content, which slows down the release of sugar into the blood stream.

Good Day Sunshine

Quick to make and very low in calories, the Good Day Sunshine smoothie is refreshing and delicious. It's an ideal way to get the day off to a good start.

Ingredients
1/2 peach
1/2 orange
1/2 apricot
1 tomato
3/4 cup crushed ice

Preparation
Place the ingredients in the blender, with the ice going in last, and blend until smooth.

Nutrition
Calories – 79g
Fibre – 4g
Fat – 0g
Protein – 2g
Carbohydrate – 16g

Ingredient Spotlight - Tomatoes
Because of their low carbohydrate content, tomatoes can play a big role in controlling blood sugar levels. Being low in carbohydrates means they are low in calories as well, and so can help diabetics to lose weight.

Tomatoes are also a rich source of antioxidants and help restore the body's oxidative balance. This can reduce the risk of complications associated with adult diabetes.

High & Low

High in fibre and low in sugar, celery is perfect for diabetics. With an apple for vitamins and a peach for potassium, this super smoothie is just what the doctor ordered.

Ingredients

2 celery sticks

1 apple

1 peach

1 tablespoon chia seeds

3/4 cup water

Preparation

Place the ingredients in the blender and blend until nice and smooth.

Nutrition

Calories – 195g

Fibre – 11g

Fat – 3g

Protein – 4g

Carbohydrate – 40g

Ingredient Spotlight - Celery

Celery is high in fibre, which improves sugar metabolism and increases insulin sensitivity. This helps to control blood sugar levels and reduce insulin.

Celery is also high in vitamin K, which can reduce the risk of developing type 2 diabetes considerably. This is due to vitamin K's ability to reduce systemic inflammation, which improves the body's ability to use insulin.

The Green One

Loaded with essential nutrients and with minimal carbohydrates, The Green One is tailor-made for the diabetic.

Ingredients
1/2 cup spinach
1/2 cup cauliflower
1/2 cup broccoli
1/2 cucumber
1 kiwi
1 cup water

Preparation
Blend the spinach, cauliflower, broccoli and water first. Then add the cucumber and the kiwi and blend again until smooth.

Nutrition
Calories – 91g
Fibre – 5g
Fat – 0.5g
Protein – 4g
Carbohydrate – 19g

Ingredient Spotlight - Broccoli

People with diabetes are up to five times more likely to develop cardiovascular diseases such as heart attacks and strokes. This is due to damaged blood vessels and the formation of plaque that blocks the flow of blood.

Broccoli contains a compound called sulforaphane that encourages the production of enzymes, which protect blood vessels and reduce the number of molecules that can damage cells.

Steady Eddie

With blood sugar-stabilizing oats, this wholesome smoothie will keep your blood sugar level under control all day.

Ingredients
1/4 cup oats
1/2 cup watermelon
1/2 cup papaya
1 tomato
1 cup water

Preparation
Put all the ingredients in the blender and blend until smooth and creamy.

Nutrition
Calories – 117g
Fibre – 3g
Fat – 1g
Protein – 3g
Carbohydrate – 26g

Ingredient Spotlight - Oats

Oats is a heart-healthy food that lowers the levels of bad cholesterol (LDL). This is important for the diabetic as diabetes is known to raise bad cholesterol, which of course can lead to heart disease and strokes.

Oats is also high in fibre that slows down digestion, which results in a lower and steadier blood sugar level.

Go Nuts

Deliciously wholesome with a low carbohydrate count, this smoothie offers plenty of fibre and a large amount of protein. Plus, it tastes just great.

Ingredients

1/2 cup kale
1 small passion fruit
1 apple
1/3 cup almonds
1 cup water

Preparation

Blend the almonds with the water first. Then add the rest of the ingredients and blend again until smooth.

Nutrition

Calories – 391g
Fibre – 11.5g
Fat – 25g
Protein – 11g
Carbohydrate – 39g

Ingredient Spotlight - Almonds

Almonds can help people with type 2 diabetes to regulate the amount of glucose and cholesterol in their blood. They do this by reducing after-meal rises in blood sugar and insulin levels.

Regular almond consumption also helps increase the level of good cholesterol (HDL) and reduce the level of bad cholesterol (LDL).

Get Up and Go

Created for diabetics who need plenty of energy, this powerhouse of a smoothie certainly delivers.

Ingredients

1 sweet potato

1/2 cup cranberries

1/2 cup asparagus

1/2 inch piece of root ginger

1 lime

1 cup almond milk

Preparation

Cut the sweet potato into small chunks before adding to the blender. Peel the lime and add whole. Then add the rest of the ingredients and blend until smooth.

Nutrition

Calories – 239g

Fibre – 12g

Fat – 2.5g

Protein – 4g

Carbohydrate – 49g

Ingredient Spotlight - Asparagus

Regular consumption of asparagus helps keep blood sugar levels under control and boosts the body's production of insulin.

Asparagus is also a good source of antioxidants, which help remove harmful free radicals from the body. This offers protection against cancer, neuro-degenerative diseases and viral infections.

CHAPTER 11

Smoothies For Extra Energy

Your body doesn't run on fresh air – it needs energy, and that energy comes from the foods you eat. Unfortunately, much of the food consumed in the typical western diet doesn't actually provide that much of it. For this read sugary foods and drinks, pasta, bread, ready meals and the like.

Foods of this type work in two ways - neither of them to your benefit. Firstly, they contain toxins and other undesirable stuff that the body has to deal with – this requires energy that is effectively lost as a result. Secondly, they contain highly refined sugars that burn quickly and so do not provide any long-term energy.

The solution is to eat plenty of plant-based foods that provide the fibre, carbohydrates (including complex sugars), and protein that provide the energy you need. Smoothies are an easy way to do this.

On a High

This smoothie combines high-alkaline ingredients that will not only dramatically boost your energy level, but also maintain it by keeping your blood-sugar level high.

Ingredients

1/4 cup spinach

1/4 cup kale

1/4 cup avocado

1/4 cup cashew nuts

1 tablespoon coconut oil

1 cup water

Preparation

Soak the cashews for at least 30 minutes beforehand - overnight ideally. Put the spinach and kale in the blender first. Then add the rest of the ingredients and blend until smooth.

Nutrition

Calories – 472g

Fibre – 4.5g

Fat – 37g

Protein – 8g

Carbohydrate – 17g

Ingredient Spotlight - Cashew Nuts

High in mineral content, particularly copper, cashew nuts help to maintain the balance of minerals needed for optimum health. Their copper content helps the body to create new red blood cells and generate energy.

Citrus Punch

The Citrus Punch is a simple and quick-to-make smoothie that tastes delicious and is guaranteed to keep you going all day. Everybody should try this one.

Ingredients
1/2 cup pineapple
1/2 grapefruit
1 small orange
1/2 lemon
3/4 cup crushed ice

Preparation
Cut the pineapple into chunks before adding to the blender. Peel the lemon and add with the other ingredients. Blend until the mixture is smooth.

Nutrition
Calories – 140g
Fibre – 6g
Fat – 0g
Protein – 2g
Carbohydrate – 36g

Ingredient Spotlight - Grapefruit
Grapefruit is well known for its ability to boost energy. It contains a compound called nootkatone that improves the way the body metabolises, i.e. generates energy from nutrients.

Grapefruit is also an excellent source of vitamins C and A. Not only that, it provides a good amount of fibre, which benefits the body's digestive system.

Energy In a Glass

The ingredients in this powerhouse of a smoothie are chosen for their ability to not just give you energy, but loads of it.

Ingredients
1/2 apple
1/2 orange
1/2 cup watermelon
1/2 cup blueberries
1/2 lime
2 or 3 mint leaves
3/4 cup water

Preparation
Peel the lime before adding it to the blender with the rest of the ingredients. Blend until smooth.

Nutrition
Calories – 151g
Fibre – 7g
Fat – 0.5g
Protein – 2.5g
Carbohydrate – 40g

Ingredient Spotlight - Asparagus
Apples are great sources of soluble fibre, vitamin C and antioxidants called polyphenols. They are also rich in fructose - the predominant sugar found in fruits which, quite literally, gives your body energy to burn.

Stay All Day

This smoothie is both delicious and refreshing. With pineapple, banana, coconut and papaya, it is also loaded with energy-rich nutrients that will keep you energized from morning to night.

Ingredients

1/2 cup pineapple
1/2 cup papaya
1 banana
2 celery sticks
1/2 cup coconut water

Preparation

Place all the ingredients in the blender and blend until nice and smooth.

Nutrition

Calories – 211g
Fibre – 8g
Fat – 1g
Protein – 4g
Carbohydrate – 52g

Ingredient Spotlight - Pineapples

Pineapple is an excellent source of vitamin C and the mineral manganese, both of which help protect against cell damage caused by free radicals. Manganese is also essential in the production of a number of enzymes that the body needs in order to generate energy.

Bop to the Beet

This vegetable-based smoothie is quite literally brimming with fibre, slow-burning carbohydrates, minerals and antioxidants. The energy you get from it will keep you on fire.

Ingredients

1/2 beet

1/2 cup mushroom

1/2 cup spinach

1 carrot

1 tomato

1 cup unsweetened almond milk

Preparation

Place the spinach in the blender first. Then add the rest of the ingredients and blend until smooth.

Nutrition

Calories – 123g

Fibre – 6g

Fat – 2.5g

Protein – 4g

Carbohydrate – 24.5g

Ingredient Spotlight - Mushrooms

Mushrooms provide a huge amount of iron, which is essential for the transportation of oxygen within the bloodstream. When the body's organs are deprived of oxygen, we feel tired and lethargic.

Iron Man

The Iron Man is a tasty combination of nutrient-rich peaches, raspberries, banana, raisins and yoghurt. This smoothie has a high iron content courtesy of the peach and raisins.

Ingredients

1 peach
1/2 cup raspberries
1/4 cup raisins
1 banana
1 cup low-fat yoghurt

Preparation

Place all the ingredients in the blender and blend until smooth and creamy.

Nutrition

Calories – 408g
Fibre – 10g
Fat – 3.5g
Protein – 11g
Carbohydrate – 90g

Ingredient Spotlight - Peaches

As with mushrooms, peaches are rich in iron that plays an important role in the formation of red blood cells and the transportation of oxygen from the lungs to the rest of the body.

Peaches are rich in beta-carotene, which helps in maintaining healthy eyesight, and the prevention of various eye diseases such as xerophthalmia and blindness.

Cucumber Cooler

A wholesome and energizing mix of vegetable and fruit, the Cucumber Cooler can be taken at breakfast to get you off to a great start or, indeed, whenever you need a boost.

Ingredients

1/2 cup watermelon

1/2 cucumber

1/2 apple

1/2 fennel

1 kiwi

1/2 cup water

Preparation

Place the kale in the blender first. Then add the other ingredients and blend until smooth.

Nutrition

Calories – 139g

Fibre – 9g

Fat – 1g

Protein – 5g

Carbohydrates – 34g

Ingredient Spotlight - Cucumbers

Cucumbers are a great source of vitamins. These include vitamin K, vitamin C and, more importantly for people needing energy, vitamin B5. This helps the body convert carbohydrates into glucose, which it then uses to produce energy.

Fly High

Rich in a variety of important nutrients, this vegetable smoothie will keep your energy level at a constant high throughout the day and enable you to deal with whatever may come your way.

Ingredients

1/2 cup watercress

1/2 bell pepper

2 celery sticks

1 tomato

1 onion

3/4 cup water

Preparation

Place the watercress in the blender first. Then add the rest of the ingredients and blend until smooth.

Nutrition

Calories – 99g

Fibre – 6g

Fat – 0g

Protein – 4.5g

Carbohydrates – 21g

Ingredient Spotlight - Watercress

Rich in the B vitamins, beta-carotene, magnesium and potassium, watercress helps to suppress the damage caused by free radicals in the body after high-intensity exercise.

It does this by raising levels of important antioxidant vitamins that enable the body to retain the health-giving benefits of the exercise.

Potato & Pecan

Sweet potatoes provide an excellent base for an energy smoothie. Combined with creamy banana, pecans and ginger, they produce a slightly sweet, spicy and extremely tasty energy drink.

Ingredients

1 uncooked sweet potato

2 tablespoons pecan nuts

1 banana

1/2 inch piece of root ginger

1 teaspoon cinnamon

1 cup unsweetened almond milk

Preparation

Peel the potato and cut into small chunks. Add the pecans and almond milk and blend. Then add the banana and ginger and blend again until smooth.

Nutrition

Calories – 375g

Fibre – 11g

Fat – 13g

Protein – 5.5g

Carbohydrates – 64g

Ingredient Spotlight - Sweet Potatoes

Sweet potatoes have a low glycemic index, which means they release sugar slowly into the bloodstream. As a result, your energy level is not only kept steady but is also maintained over a longer period than would otherwise be the case.

CHAPTER 12

Smoothies For Bones and Teeth

Just as with every other part of the human body, bones and teeth require specific nutrients in order to grow and stay healthy. These include vitamin D, which helps absorb calcium from food; and vitamin C, which synthesizes collagen and gives your bones tensile strength.

Also required is calcium, phosphorus, magnesium, potassium, manganese, zinc, iron and silica. Plus, there are healthy fats and cholesterol that the body needs in order to absorb these nutrients.

Calcium is probably the most important nutrient of all, and the smoothies in this chapter will ensure you get a plentiful supply of it. This alone will help keep your bones and teeth in good condition.

The Bone Builder

A lovely green smoothie that contains a good number of the nutrients your body needs in order to build and maintain strong, healthy bones.

Ingredients
1/2 cup broccoli
1/2 cup spinach
1/4 cup avocado
1 parsnip
1 tablespoon sesame seeds
3/4 cup low-fat milk

Preparation
Blend the sesame seeds with the milk first. Then add the other ingredients and blend again until smooth.

Nutrition
Calories – 260g
Fibre – 7g
Fat – 12.0g
Protein – 11g
Carbohydrate – 30g

Ingredient Spotlight - Avocados

Avocados contains a number of vitamins that include B vitamins, vitamin K and vitamin E. The latter is extremely important with regard to bones as it ensures they grow properly and that bone density is maintained in later life.

Avocados also contain carotenoids such as zeaxanthin and lutein, which are associated with a reduced risk of osteoarthritis.

Black & Blue

The Black and Blue smoothie is a delicious and highly refreshing drink that comes with the added benefit of being rich in the calcium that your bones and teeth require.

Ingredients

1/2 cup rhubarb
1/2 cup blueberries
1/4 cup goji berries
1 tablespoon of chia seeds
1/2 cup low-fat yoghurt
2 or 3 ice cubes

Preparation

Place all the smoothie ingredients in the blender with the ice cubes going in last. Blend until smooth.

Nutrition

Calories – 310g
Fibre – 14g
Fat – 4g
Protein – 12g
Carbohydrate – 58g

Ingredient Spotlight - Chia Seeds

Chia seeds contain more calcium than most dairy products (worth remembering, perhaps!). In fact, just two tablespoons provides 20 percent of the recommended daily amount for adults.

The seeds are also high in magnesium, phosphorus and protein - all of which are essential for bone health.

Molar Madness

An unfortunate side effect of eating too much refined sugar is tooth decay. The ingredients in this smoothie work well together to help strengthen teeth weakened by cavities.

Ingredients

1 banana

1 tablespoon cod liver oil

1 teaspoon ghee

1 teaspoon honey

1 cup green tea

Preparation

Brew the green tea first then add to the blender with the other ingredients. The honey is optional but does give this smoothie a nicer taste.

Nutrition

Calories – 291g

Fibre – 3g

Fat – 19g

Protein – 1.5g

Carbohydrate – 44g

Ingredient Spotlight - Ghee

Ghee (clarified butter) contains a fat-soluble vitamin called K2. This vitamin is essential in enabling the body to utilize minerals such as calcium.

Correct levels of vitamin K2 help to protect against tooth decay, supports the growth and development of bones, and helps to prevent calcification of the arteries (a process known as atherosclerosis).

Smile, You're On Camera

Another one for the teeth, this smoothie will have you smiling your head off and not just because of the great taste. Full of calcium and fibre, it kills mouth bacteria and helps whiten teeth.

Ingredients

1 apple
1/4 cup avocado
2 kiwis
2 or 3 mint leaves
1/2 cup water

Preparation

Place all the ingredients in the blender. Blend until smooth and creamy.

Nutrition

Calories – 251g
Fibre – 11.5g
Fat – 8g
Protein – 3.5g
Carbohydrate – 49g

Ingredient Spotlight - Apples

The fibre-rich flesh in an apple acts like a scrubbing brush on your tongue, teeth and gums. This helps remove plaque and stains from the teeth and helps to whiten them.

Furthermore, apples are mildly acidic in nature and have a astringent quality that also helps to remove plaque.

Chew On This

The Chew On This smoothie achieves its objective of healthy teeth thanks to its high manganese content. This one is not just for the teeth however, it is equally effective for bone strength.

Ingredients

1/2 cup pineapple

1 apricot

1 orange

4 dates

3/4 cup coconut water

Preparation

Cut the pineapple, apricot and orange into chunks before placing in the blender. Then add the dates and coconut water and blend until smooth.

Nutrition

Calories – 252g

Fibre – 7.5g

Fat – 0.5g

Protein – 4g

Carbohydrate – 64g

Ingredient Spotlight - Pineapple

Pineapple contains nearly 75 percent of the recommended daily amount of manganese. This mineral is essential in the development of teeth, bones and connective tissue.

Pineapple is also high in vitamin C, which the body needs for collagen synthesis. Collagen is the main structural protein in the body for a number of things, one of which is bone strength.

Anyone For Tea?

This tasty smoothie provides a number of compounds all of which have beneficial effects on the health of bones and teeth.

Ingredients

1/2 cup asparagus

1/2 cup butternut squash

1 celery stick

1 carrot

1/2 apple

1 cup green tea

Preparation

Blend the celery, carrot and apple first. Then add the kale and the cup of green tea and blend again until smooth.

Nutrition

Calories – 100g

Fibre – 6g

Fat – 0g

Protein – 3.5g

Carbohydrate – 24g

Ingredient Spotlight   Green Tea

Green tea protects oral health by preventing plaque build-up. This is due to the polyphenols it contains that either destroy or suppress plaque bacteria. The result is a significant slowdown of their growth, which reduces the quantity of acids they produce.

Green tea is also thought to reverse the damage caused by chronic inflammation. This damage can lead to bone loss over time and may increase the risk of osteoporosis.

Blind Date

This super smoothie is a real powerhouse. The raspberries alone provide magnesium, calcium and manganese, all of which are essential for healthy bones and teeth.

Ingredients

1/2 cup dates

1/2 cup raspberries

1/4 cup avocado

1 tablespoon powdered acai berries

1/2 inch piece root ginger

1/2 cup unsweetened almond milk

Preparation

Put the ingredients in the blender and blend until smooth and creamy.

Nutrition

Calories – 397g

Fibre – 19g

Fat – 10g

Protein – 4.5g

Carbohydrate – 83g

Ingredient Spotlight - Dates

Dates are rich in selenium, manganese, copper and magnesium. These compounds are all essential for keeping bones healthy and preventing conditions such as osteoporosis. The high sugar content of dates is perhaps not so good for teeth though!

Dates are also rich in fluorine. This is a mineral that fights tooth decay, which is why it is added to toothpaste in the form of fluoride.

Peach Perfect

Another all-rounder that is good for both bones and teeth. A lot of the goodness in this one comes from the peach, an important component of which is phosphorous.

Ingredients
1 peach
1 banana
1/2 cup cherries
1 cup low-fat yoghurt

Preparation
Put the ingredients in the blender and blend until smooth and creamy.

Nutrition
Calories – 305g
Fibre – 6g
Fat – 3g
Protein – 10g
Carbohydrate – 65g

Ingredient Spotlight - Peaches

Peaches contain phosphorous which, together with calcium, helps to strengthen bones and teeth. It also helps to prevent a number of bone diseases, such as osteoporosis.

The high vitamin C content in peaches works to strengthen the jaw bones and gums, which is obviously important for the teeth.

Tooth Wisdom

Our last smoothie in this chapter is an ideal one for teeth and gums. This fang-friendly concoction includes cranberries, which are well known for their ability to prevent tooth decay.

Ingredients

1/2 cup kale

1/2 apple

1/2 cup cranberries

1 celery stick

1/4 cup almonds

1 cup low-fat milk

Preparation

Blend the almonds with the milk first. Then add the kale followed by the rest of the ingredients. Blend again until smooth.

Nutrition

Calories – 416g

Fibre – 9g

Fat – 21g

Protein – 17g

Carbohydrate – 42g

Ingredient Spotlight - Cranberries

Cranberries contain a compound called proanthocyanidine. This helps to stop harmful bacteria from adhering to teeth and eventually causing tooth decay and cavities.

It also helps to prevent the growth of plaque, thus preventing periodontal (gum) disease.

CHAPTER 13

Smoothies For General Good Health

So far we've concentrated on smoothies aimed at various parts of the body. In this chapter, we'll broaden our approach by taking a look at smoothies that are good for you generally.

These are perfect for those of you who don't have any specific health issues and want to keep it that way. Most of these drinks will have system-wide benefits and taking them on a regular basis is one of the best ways available to you of keeping your body fit and healthy. Take them and, if it isn't already, it soon will be.

Tropical Treat

This super smoothie has more health benefits than we have room to mention. Suffice to say, it is rich in protein, healthy fats, potassium and vitamin C. This is one you simply have to try.

Ingredients

1 banana

1/2 avocado

1 passion fruit

1 kiwi

1 cup coconut water

Preparation

Cut the various fruits into chunks before adding to the blender. Add the coconut water and blend until smooth.

Nutrition

Calories – 343g

Fibre – 14g

Fat – 8.5g

Protein – 6g

Carbohydrate – 54g

Ingredient Spotlight - Avocados

Nutrition-wise, these fruit are at the head of the pack. Packed with fibre, just one avocado contains 36 percent of the daily requirement of vitamin K, 30 percent of the folate, and 20 percent each of the daily requirements of vitamin B5, vitamin B6, vitamin C and potassium.

Basically, every part of the body will benefit from eating avocado. While they do have a very high fat content – 32 percent - these are actually heart-friendly fats that you can eat quite safely.

Blueberry Blitz

The Blueberry Blitz is a deliciously smooth and creamy drink thanks to the banana and almond butter. It is also extremely good for you as it contains a shed-load of nutrients.

Ingredients

1/2 cup blueberries

1/2 cup asparagus

1/2 cup coconut meat

1 banana

1 tablespoon almond butter

1 cup low-fat milk

Preparation

Place all ingredients into the blender and blend until smooth and creamy.

Nutrition

Calories – 472g

Fibre – 11g

Fat – 26g

Protein – 17.5g

Carbohydrate – 62g

Ingredient Spotlight - Coconut

Coconut is highly nutritious and rich in fibre, vitamins C, E, B1, B3, B5 and B6; and minerals including iron, selenium, sodium, calcium, magnesium and phosphorous.

Coconut does contain significant amounts of saturated fat. However, this is not the same as the saturated fat found in animals, and is considered to be much healthier.

Minty Mango

The Minty Mango is a simple and quick-to-make smoothie that is both nutritious and refreshing.

Ingredients

1/2 cup mango
1/2 cup pineapple
1 cup coconut water
3 or 4 mint leaves
2 ice cubes

Preparation

Cut the pineapple and mango into chunks. Then add to the blender with the coconut water and mint leaves. Add the ice cubes last and blend until smooth.

Nutrition

Calories – 160g
Fibre – 5.5g
Fat – 0.5g
Protein – 1.5g
Carbohydrate – 37g

Ingredient Spotlight - Mangoes

Mangos are one of the most consumed fruits in the world and provide a range of health benefits. They contain an antioxidant called zeaxanthin, which is thought to play a protective role in eye health and prevent damage from macular degeneration.

Because of their high fibre and water content, mangos help to prevent constipation and promote a healthy digestive tract.

Rhubarb & Apple

This smoothie is absolutely loaded with fibre, not to mention a wide range of nutrients that will benefit most parts of the body in one way or another.

Ingredients

1/2 cup rhubarb
1/2 apple
1 celery stick
1 tomato
3/4 cup water
2 or 3 ice cubes

Preparation

Chop the ingredients into chunks. Add to the blender with the water and ice and blend until smooth.

Nutrition

Calories – 101g
Fibre – 4g
Fat – 0g
Protein – 2g
Carbohydrate – 21g

Ingredient Spotlight - Rhubarb

A much underrated food, rhubarb provides a whole range of health benefits. These include maintenance of the digestive system due to the high fibre content.

Rhubarb is also rich in vitamin K, which has a significant role in the body's neurological functions. For example, it can stimulate cognitive activity thereby helping to delay, or even prevent, the onset of Alzheimer's disease.

Cherrylicious

Cherrylicious by name and delicious by nature, the ingredients in this not-to-miss smoothie will help you to work, rest and play.

Ingredients
1/2 cup cherries
1/2 cup red grapes
1/2 cup spinach
1/4 avocado
1 cup unsweetened almond milk
1 sprig rosemary

Preparation
Place all the ingredients in the blender, with the spinach going in first, and blend until smooth.

Nutrition
Calories – 227g
Fibre – 6g
Fat – 9g
Protein – 3g
Carbohydrate – 36g

Ingredient Spotlight - Cherries

Cherries provide a range of health benefits. They are high in fibre, vitamin C, carotenoids and anthocyanins - all of which may help play a role in cancer prevention.

Also present in cherries is melatonin, an antioxidant that reduces inflammation and plays a vital role in sleep and body regeneration.

Ginger & Blackberry

The Ginger and Blackberry is a healthy, delicious and satisfying smoothie that will fill you up and keep you away from the refrigerator.

Ingredients

1/2 cup blackberries
1/2 cucumber
1/2 apple
1/4 cup oats
1/2 inch piece of root ginger
1 cup fresh pineapple juice

Preparation

Place all the ingredients in the blender and blend until nice and smooth.

Nutrition

Calories – 284g
Fibre – 13g
Fat – 2g
Protein – 4g
Carbohydrate – 66g

Ingredient Spotlight - Blackberries

Blackberries are rich in vitamin C. They are also an excellent source of both soluble and insoluble fibre. Plus, they contain a good amount of minerals such as potassium, manganese, magnesium and copper.

The latter is required for bone metabolism and the production of white and red blood cells.

Just Nuts

Legumes are nutritional powerhouses, so this smoothie will keep you going all day.

Ingredients
1/2 cup watermelon
1/2 cup coconut meat
1 banana
1 tablespoon peanut butter
1/2 cup unsweetened almond milk
2 or 3 basil leaves

Preparation
Place all the ingredients in the blender and blend until smooth and creamy.

Nutrition
Calories – 391g
Fibre – 8.5g
Fat – 23.5g
Protein – 7g
Carbohydrate – 46g

Ingredient Spotlight - Peanut Butter

Peanut butter is a high calorie food due to the amount of fat it contains. However, the fat is the mono-unsaturated type that is actually good for the heart.

It is rich in both fibre and protein – these fill you up and keep you feeling full for longer. Also present in peanut butter is the antioxidant vitamin E, bone-building magnesium, muscle-friendly potassium, and immunity-boosting vitamin B6.

Pearshaped

Containing three recognized superfoods – kale, asparagus and chia seeds, this smoothie is quite literally packed with all-round goodness. The pear helps to alleviate the 'veggie' taste.

Ingredients

1/2 cup kale

1/2 cup asparagus

1 pear

1 tablespoon chia seeds

3/4 cup water

Preparation

Blend the chia seeds with the water first. Then add the kale, pear and asparagus and blend again until smooth.

Nutrition

Calories – 176g

Fibre – 11g

Fat – 3.5g

Protein – 3g

Carbohydrate – 35g

Ingredient Spotlight - Asparagus

Asparagus is one of the best natural sources of folate. Adequate folate intake is extremely important during periods of rapid growth such as pregnancy, infancy and adolescence. Folate may also help to protect against colon, stomach, pancreatic and cervical cancers.

Asparagus is also a good source of potassium, fibre and thiamin, plus vitamins A, B6 and C.

It Figgers

The It Figgers smoothie is for health-freaks who also happen to have a sweet tooth. This one will put a smile on your face and keep it there all day long.

Ingredients
1/2 mango
4 figs
4 dates
1 banana
3/4 cup coconut water

Preparation
Cut the mango into chunks. Then add to the blender with the other ingredients and blend until smooth.

Nutrition
Calories – 502g
Fibre – 13.5g
Fat – 2g
Protein – 9g
Carbohydrate – 125g

Ingredient Spotlight - Figs
Figs have a high fibre content. This helps promote regular bowel function and prevents constipation and diarrhoea.

Figs are rich in calcium, which is one of the most important components in strengthening bones, and thus reducing the risk of osteoporosis. They also contain a good amount of phosphorus, which encourages bone formation.

Nutritional Value of Fresh Fruit

	Calories	Fiber	Fat	Protein	Carbs
Apple - 1 medium	95	4.5g	0.5g	0.5g	25g
Apricot - 1 medium	14	0.5g	0g	0.5g	3g
Banana - 1 medium	105	3g	0.5g	1.5g	27g
Blackberry - 1 cup	62	7.5g	0.5g	2g	14g
Blueberry - 1 cup	83	3.5g	0.5g	1g	21g
Cherry - 1 cup	74	2.5g	0g	1g	19g
Coconut meat - 1 cup	283	7g	27g	2.5g	12g
Cranberry - 1 cup	60	4g	0g	0g	10g
Dates - 1 cup	495	15g	0g	4g	133g
Elderberry - 1 cup	106	10g	0.5g	1g	27g
Figs - 1 cup	492	20g	2g	6g	127g
Grapes - 1 cup	110	1g	0g	1g	27g
Grapefruit - 1 medium	82	3g	0g	1.5g	20g
Guava - 1 medium	61	5g	1g	2.5g	13g
Kiwi - 1 medium	42	2g	0.5g	1g	10g
Lemon - 1 medium	17	1.5g	0g	0.5g	5.5g
Lime - 1 medium	20	2g	0g	0.5g	7g
Mango - 1 medium	145	3.5g	0.5g	1g	35g
Mulberry - 1 cup	60	2.5g	0.5g	2g	14g
Orange - 1 medium	62	3g	0g	1g	15g
Papaya - 1 cup	60	2.5g	0.5g	0.5g	16g
Passion Fruit - 1 med	5	0.5g	0.5g	0.5g	1g
Peach - 1 medium	38	1.5g	0g	1g	9g
Pear - 1 medium	96	5g	0g	0.5g	25g
Plum - 1 medium	20	0.5g	0g	0.5g	5g
Pineapple - 1 cup	82	2.5g	0g	1g	21g
Pomegranate - 1 med	100	1g	0.5g	1g	26g
Raspberry - 1 cup	64	8g	1g	1.5g	15g
Rhubarb - 1 cup	26	2g	0g	1g	5.5g
Strawberry - 1 cup	49	3g	0.5g	1g	12g
Watermelon - 1 cup	45	0.5g	0g	1g	11g

Nutritional Value of Dried Fruit

	Calories	Fiber	Fat	Protein	Carbs
Apple - 1 cup	240	6g	0g	1g	50g
Apricots - 1 cup	310	9.5g	0.5g	4.5g	82g
Cranberries - 1 cup	520	8g	0g	0g	136g
Dates - 1 cup	493	15g	0g	4g	133g
Figs - 1 cup	490	20g	2g	6g	127g
Goji Berries - 1 cup	300	2g	3g	18g	60g
Prunes - 1 cup	408	12g	0.5g	3.5g	109g
Raisins - 1 cup	436	5g	1g	4g	115g
Sultanas - 1 cup	656	4.5g	0g	4.5g	154g

Nutritional Value of Fruit Juices

	Calories	Fiber	Fat	Protein	Carbs
Apple - 1 cup	117	0g	0.5g	0g	29g
Beetroot - 1 cup	96	0g	0g	3g	21g
Carrot - 1 cup	80	0g	0g	2g	17g
Cranberry - 1 cup	110	0g	0g	0g	28g
Grapefruit - 1 cup	96	0g	0g	1g	23g
Lemon - 1 tablespoon	3	0g	0g	0g	1g
Lime - 1 tablespoon	5	0g	0g	0g	1.5g
Orange - 1 cup	112	0.5g	0.5g	1.5g	26g
Pineapple - 1 cup	120	0g	0g	0g	31g
Pomegranate - 1 cup	100	0g	0g	0g	20g
Prune - 1cup	180	2.5g	0g	1.5g	45g
Tomato - 1 cup	41	1g	0g	2g	10g
Coconut water - 1 cup	46	2.5g	0.5g	1.5g	9g

Nutritional Value of Vegetables

	Calories	Fiber	Fat	Protein	Carbs
Artichoke - 1 medium	60	7g	0g	4g	13g
Asparagus - 1 cup	27	3g	0g	3g	5g
Avocado - 1 medium	289	12g	26.5g	3.5g	15g
Beetroot - 1 medium	35	2.5g	0g	1.5g	8g
Broccoli - 1 cup	31	2.5g	0.5g	2.5g	6g
Brussels Sprouts - 1 cup	38	3.5g	0.5g	3g	8g
Cabbage - 1 cup	22	2g	0g	1g	5g
Carrots - 1 medium	25	1.5g	0g	0.5g	6g
Cauliflower - 1 cup	25	2.5g	0g	2g	5.5g
Celery - 1 stalk	6	0.5g	0g	0.5g	1g
Courgette - 1 medium	40	2g	1g	3.5g	5g
Cucumber - 1 medium	24	1.5g	0.5g	1g	4.5g
Eggplant - 1 medium	21	3g	0.5g	1g	5g
Fennel - 1 medium	73	7g	0.5g	3g	17g
Ginger - 1 teaspoon	1.5	1g	0g	0g	1g
Green Beans - 1 cup	34	3.5g	0g	2g	8g
Kale - 1 cup	33	1g	1g	0.5g	7g
Lettuce - 1 cup	10	0g	0g	1g	2g
Mushrooms - 1 cup	15	1g	0g	2g	2g
Onion - 1 medium	47	2.5g	0g	1.5g	10g
Parsnip - 1 cup	100	6g	0.5g	1.5g	24g
Pepper - 1 medium	30	2g	0g	1g	8g
Potato - 1 medium	164	4.5g	0g	4g	37g
Pumpkin - 1 medium	30g	0.5g	0g	1g	7.5g
Radish - 1 cup	13	1g	0g	1g	4g
Spinach - 1 cup	7	1g	0g	1g	1g
Squash - 1 cup	18	1g	0g	1.5g	4g
Sweet Potato - 1 med	112	4g	0g	3g	26g
Tomato - 1 medium	22	1.5g	0g	1g	5g
Turnip - 1 medium	34	2g	0g	1g	8g
Watercress - 1 cup	7	0.5g	0g	1g	0g
Zucchini - 1 medium	32	2g	0.5g	2.5g	6.5g

Nutritional Value of Nuts

	Calories	Fiber	Fat	Protein	Carbs
Almonds - 1 cup	823	17.5g	71g	30g	31g
Brazil - 1 cup	920	10g	93g	20g	17g
Cashews - 1 cup	960	4g	76g	28g	44g
Chestnuts - 1 cup	210	2g	2g	4g	44g
Coconut - 1 cup	490	14g	50g	7g	8g
Hazelnuts - 1 cup	720	8g	72g	16g	16g
Macadamia - 1 cup	961	11g	101g	10.5g	18.5g
Peanuts - 1 cup	825	12g	71g	38g	24g
Pecans - 1 cup	760	4g	80g	12g	16g
Pistachios - 1 cup	740	12g	52g	24g	36g
Walnuts - 1 cup	800	8g	80g	20g	16g

Nutritional Value of Seeds

	Calories	Fiber	Fat	Protein	Carbs
Chia - 1 tablespoon	67	5.5g	4.5g	3g	0.5g
Flax - 1 tablespoon	37	2g	2g	1.5g	2g
Hemp - 1 tablespoon	57	0.5g	4.5g	3.5g	0.5g
Linseeds - 1 tablespoon	49	2.5g	4g	1.5g	2.5g
Poppy - 1 tablespoon	47	1g	4g	1.5g	2g
Pumpkin - 1 tablespoon	56	0.5g	5g	3g	1g
Sesame - 1 tablespoon	52	1g	4.5g	1.5g	2g
Sunflower - 1 tablespoon	47	1g	4g	1.5g	2g

Nutritional Value of Pulses

	Calories	Fiber	Fat	Protein	Carbs
Blackeyed peas - 1 cup	200	8g	4g	12g	34g
Black beans - 1 cup	240	12g	1g	14g	46g
Broad beans - 1 cup	160	8g	0.5g	10g	28g
Butter beans - 1 cup	200	10g	0g	10g	38g
Chickpeas - 1 cup	210	7g	3g	11g	34g
Green Peas - 1 cup	117	7.5g	0.5g	8g	21g
Lentils - 1 cup	320	44g	0g	40g	80g
Mung beans - 1 cup	600	33g	1.5g	49g	110g
Pinto beans - 1 cup	670	30g	2.5g	41g	120g
Kidney beans - 1 cup	216	15.5g	0g	14g	43g
Soya beans - 1 cup	290	12g	14.5g	28g	10g
Split Peas - 1 cup	440	48g	0g	40g	112g

Nutritional Value of Misc

	Calories	Fiber	Fat	Protein	Carbs
Almond milk - 1 cup	60	0.5g	2.5g	0.5g	8g
Almond butter - 1 tbsp	102	0.5g	9g	3.5g	3g
Honey - 1 tbsp	70	0.5g	0g	0g	17g
Soya milk - 1 cup	132	1.5g	4.5g	8g	15.5g
Low-fat yoghurt - 1 cup	125	0g	2.5g	7g	19g
Low-fat milk - 1 cup	110	0g	2.5g	9g	13g
Protein powder - 1 tbsp	110	0g	1.5g	23g	1g
Peanut butter - 1 tbsp	94	1g	8g	4g	3g
Cinnamon - 1 teaspoon	6	1g	0g	0g	4g
Turmeric - 1 tbsp	24	1.5g	0.5g	1g	120g
Oats - 1 cup	166	4g	3.5g	6g	28g
Cod liver oil - 1 tbsp	135	0g	15g	0g	0g
Olive oil - 1 tbsp	120	0g	14g	0g	0g

Conversion Charts

All the measures in this book are in US cups and spoons. Those of you who use the metric or imperial systems can use the conversion charts below to quickly convert.

Converting Liquid

US Cups	Metric	Imperial
1 cup	250 ml	8 fl oz
3/4 cup	180 ml	6 fl oz
2/3 cup	150 ml	5 fl oz
1/2 cup	120 ml	4 fl oz
1/3 cup	75 ml	2 1/2 fl oz
1/4 cup	60 ml	2 fl oz
1/8 cup	30 ml	1 fl oz
1 tablespoon	15 ml	1/2 fl oz
1 teaspoon	5 ml	1/6 fl oz

Converting Weight

The figures in the chart below are the ones needed to convert fruit and vegetables. Note that the Imperial figures are rounded up or down to the nearest 1/4 of an ounce.

US Cups	Metric	Imperial
1 cup	150 g	5 oz
3/4 cup	110 g	3 2/3 oz
2/3 cup	100 g	3 1/2 oz
1/2 cup	75 g	2 1/2 oz
1/3 cup	50 g	1 3/4 oz
1/4 cup	40 g	1 1/2 oz
1/8 cup	20 g	3/4 oz
1 tablespoon	10 g	1/3 oz
1 teaspoon	3 g	1/10 oz